T0235235

Complications in Neck Dissection

Thomas Schlieve · Waleed Zaid
Editors

Complications in Neck Dissection

A Comprehensive, Illustrated Guide

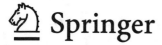 Springer

Editors
Thomas Schlieve
Division of Oral and Maxillofacial Surgery
University of Texas Southwestern
Medical Center, Texas Health Presbyterian
Hospital
Dallas, TX
USA

Waleed Zaid
Oral and Maxillofacial Surgery Department
Louisiana State University Health sciences
center – New Orleans, Our Lady of the
Lake Regional Medical center –
Baton Rouge
Baton Rouge, LA
USA

ISBN 978-3-030-62741-6   ISBN 978-3-030-62739-3   (eBook)
https://doi.org/10.1007/978-3-030-62739-3

This Springer imprint is published by the registered company Springer Nature Switzerland AG
The registered company address is: Gewerbestrasse 11, 6330 Cham, Switzerland

This book is dedicated to Cristina Bartis, my wife and partner in life. She is my best friend, my biggest supporter, my kindest critic, and my greatest love. Thank you to my mentors who encouraged me and have always supported me. "If I have seen further it is by standing on the shoulders of giants."
—Thomas Schlieve

Preface

As head and neck fellows learning the art of neck dissection, we realized an abundant number of textbooks and review articles discussing the indications for neck dissection and types of neck dissections but only short sections discussing possible complications that might arise in association with a neck dissection procedure.

We thought of creating a textbook that might shed light on these complications in greater detail and elaborate on their management. Rather than depending only on our own experience, we were fortunate to secure significant input and contribution from our distinguished authors. We made sure that the following text reflects on common and rare complications encountered in our practices and elaborated on how to prevent them.

We surely hope you enjoy reading this textbook.

Dallas, TX, USA   Thomas Schlieve
Baton Rouge, LA, USA   Waleed Zaid

Acknowledgment

First, I would like to thank my family, especially my wife Manal for the tremendous support she has shown across the years, starting from my residency carrying through fellowship and as an attending surgeon, along with our kids Yaseen and Mohammad. Also, I must thank all my faculty who contributed in my education and training, from my Canadian faculty at McGill University to my fellowship director at Boston University, Dr. Andrew Salama, and I am honored to co-author with him in one of the chapters in this textbook. Finally, I have to thank my LSUHSC family for their endless support that nourished me as faculty and allowed me to progress in my career.

New Orleans, LA, USA   Waleed Zaid

Contents

1   **Neck Dissections: History, Classification, and Indications**   1
Eric R. Carlson

2   **Complications Related to Skin Incisions, Design, and Skin Flaps**   23
Waleed Zaid, Travis Williams, Rushil Dang, and Andrew Salama

3   **Infectious Complications**   49
Lindsay L. Graves and Thomas Schlieve

4   **Complications Related to Lymphatics and Chyle Leak**   59
Waleed Zaid, Peter Park, Beomjune Kim, and Rob Laughlin

5   **Vascular Complications**   79
Anastasiya Quimby, Yoram Fleissig, and Rui Fernandes

6   **Neural Complications**   97
Moo Hyun Kim and Antonia Kolokythas

7   **Complications Related to Radical Neck Dissections
and Management of Recurrent Neck Disease** 111
Fawaz Alotaibi, Ricardo Lugo, D. David Kim, and Ghali E. Ghali

8   **Other Complications Related to Neck Dissection** 143
Roderick Y. Kim, Todd R. Wentland, Daniel A. Hammer, and
Fayette C. Williams

Index 157

Contributors

Fawaz Alotaibi, DDS Department of Oral and Maxillofacial Surgery, Head and Neck Oncology/Microvascular Reconstruction, Louisiana State University Health Sciences Center at Shreveport, Shreveport, LA, USA

Eric R. Carlson, DMD, MD, EdM, FACS Department of Oral and Maxillofacial Surgery, The University of Tennessee Graduate School of Medicine, University of Tennessee Medical Center, Knoxville, TN, USA

University of Tennessee Cancer Institute, Knoxville, TN, USA

Rushil Dang, DMD Oral and Maxillofacial Surgery Department, Boston University – School of Dentistry, Boston, MA, USA

Rui Fernandes, MD, DMD, FACS, FRCS(ed) Department of Oral and Maxillofacial Surgery, Division of Head and Neck Oncologic and Microvascular Surgery, University of Florida, Jacksonville, FL, USA

Yoram Fleissig, MD, DMD, MSc Department of Oral and Maxillofacial Surgery, Division of Head and Neck Oncologic and Microvascular Surgery, University of Florida, Jacksonville, FL, USA

Ghali E. Ghali, DDS, MD, FACS, FRCS(Ed) Department of Oral and Maxillofacial Surgery, Head and Neck Oncology, Louisiana State University Health Sciences Center at Shreveport, Shreveport, LA, USA

Lindsay L. Graves, DDS, MD Department of Oral and Maxillofacial Surgery, Parkland Memorial Hospital, Dallas, TX, USA

Daniel A. Hammer, DDS John Peter Smith Health Network, Department of Oral and Maxillofacial Surgery, Division of Maxillofacial Oncology and Reconstructive Surgery, Fort Worth, TX, USA

Beomjune Kim, DDS, MD Oral and Maxillofacial Surgery Department, Louisiana State University Health Sciences Center, New Orleans, LA, USA

Moo Hyun Kim, DDS Department of Oral and Maxillofacial Surgery, University of Rochester – Strong Memorial Hospital, Eastman Institute for Oral Health, Rochester, NY, USA

D. David Kim, DMD, MD, FACS Department of Oral and Maxillofacial Surgery, Head and Neck Oncology/Microvascular Reconstruction, Louisiana State University Health Sciences Center at Shreveport, Shreveport, LA, USA

Roderick Y. Kim, DDS MD John Peter Smith Health Network, Department of Oral and Maxillofacial Surgery, Division of Maxillofacial Oncology and Reconstructive Surgery, Fort Worth, TX, USA

Department of Surgery, Texas Christian University, Fort Worth, TX, USA

Antonia Kolokythas, DDS, MSc, MSed, FACS Department of Oral and Maxillofacial Surgery, University of Rochester – Strong Memorial Hospital, Eastman Institute for Oral Health, Rochester, NY, USA

Rob Laughlin, DDS Oral and Maxillofacial Surgery Department, Louisiana State University Health Sciences Center, New Orleans, LA, USA

Ricardo Lugo, DDS, MD Department of Oral and Maxillofacial Surgery, Head and Neck Oncology/Microvascular Reconstruction, Louisiana State University Health Sciences Center at Shreveport, Shreveport, LA, USA

Peter Park, DDS, MD Oral and Maxillofacial Surgery Department, Louisiana State University Health Sciences Center, New Orleans, LA, USA

Anastasiya Quimby, MD, DDS Department of Oral and Maxillofacial Surgery, Division of Head and Neck Oncologic and Microvascular Surgery, University of Florida, Jacksonville, FL, USA

Andrew Salama, DDS, MD, FACS Oral and Maxillofacial Surgery Department, Boston University – School of Dentistry, Boston, MA, USA

Thomas Schlieve, DDS, MD, FACS Department of Surgery, Division of Oral and Maxillofacial Surgery, UT Southwestern Medical Center, Parkland Memorial Hospital, Texas Health – Dallas Presbyterian, Dallas, TX, USA

Todd R. Wentland, DDS MD John Peter Smith Health Network, Department of Oral and Maxillofacial Surgery, Division of Maxillofacial Oncology and Reconstructive Surgery, Fort Worth, TX, USA

Travis Williams, DMD, MD Oral and Maxillofacial Surgery Department, Louisiana State University Surgery Department, New Orleans, LA, USA

Fayette C. Williams, DDS MD FACS John Peter Smith Health Network, Department of Oral and Maxillofacial Surgery, Division of Maxillofacial Oncology and Reconstructive Surgery, Fort Worth, TX, USA

Department of Surgery, Texas Christian University, Fort Worth, TX, USA

Waleed Zaid, DDS, MSc, FRCD(c) Oral and Maxillofacial Surgery Department, Louisiana State University Health Sciences Center, New Orleans, LA, USA

Neck Dissections: History, Classification, and Indications

Eric R. Carlson

History of Neck Dissections for Oral/Head and Neck Cancer

Surgical removal of the cervical lymph nodes plays a very important role in the comprehensive management of squamous cell carcinoma of the oral/head and neck anatomic region. Two of the most important aspects of the assessment of patients with these cancers, therefore, include the clinical evaluation of the lymph nodes of the neck, and the prediction of occult neck disease in the case of a clinically negative neck examination (cN0). Occult neck disease can be defined as disease that is present microscopically in cervical lymph nodes, but cannot be palpated clinically and may elude identification by special imaging studies including positron emission tomography/computed tomography (PET/CT) scans [1–3]. As such, oral/head and neck cancer patients who are statistically likely (>20%) [4] to harbor occult disease in their cervical lymph nodes are clinically staged as cN0 and should undergo elective neck dissections with the frequent and resultant histopathologic identification of metastatic disease in the cervical lymph nodes (pN+). Enhanced survival outcome assessments indicate that elective surgical removal of occult cervical lymph nodes should be executed with curative intent [5, 6].

Oral cancer is most commonly treated surgically, so it is most appropriate that the neck be simultaneously addressed surgically while reserving radiotherapy, and possibly chemotherapy for the adjuvant setting when adverse pathologic features so dictate [7]. Indeed, observing the N0 neck, only to operate the neck in the case of future, clinically apparent nodal disease, is detrimental from a survival perspective in a large majority of cases of oral squamous cell carcinoma [8]. This statement is based on the realization that salvage rates for these patients are unfavorable [9, 10].

E. R. Carlson (✉)
Department of Oral and Maxillofacial Surgery, The University of Tennessee Graduate School of Medicine, University of Tennessee Medical Center, Knoxville, TN, USA

University of Tennessee Cancer Institute, Knoxville, TN, USA
e-mail: Ecarlson@utmck.edu

© Springer Nature Switzerland AG 2021
T. Schlieve, W. Zaid (eds.), *Complications in Neck Dissection*,
https://doi.org/10.1007/978-3-030-62739-3_1

To this end, in 1839, Warren recommended removal of lymph nodes in the submandibular triangle associated with tongue cancer with the expressed intention of improving the curability of cancer at that site [11]. One of the first systematic descriptions of the importance of cervical lymph nodes in head and neck cancer was reported by Maximilian von Chelius in 1847 [12]. In 1906, a frequently quoted paper was published in *The Journal of the American Medical Association* by Dr. George Crile of the Cleveland Clinic in Ohio that reviewed the execution of neck dissection in head and neck cancer patients [13]. The paper was entitled *Excision of cancer of the head and neck – With special reference to the plan of dissection based on one hundred and thirty-two operations.* Interestingly, Crile's 1906 paper is the most commonly quoted treatise regarding this discipline and is thought to represent the first of his works on this subject, yet it was in fact his second paper published on this exercise. His first paper was published on this topic in 1905, entitled *On the surgical treatment of cancer of the head and neck – With a summary of one hundred and twenty-one operations performed upon one hundred and five patients,* in which Crile initially described an en bloc dissection of the neck [14, 15]. In the 1905 paper, Crile created an analogy between breast cancer, where regional lymph nodes are routinely excised, and head and neck cancer where a similar approach should therefore be applied. He stated that a dissection of lymph nodes of the neck is indicated whether the "glands are or are not palpable." Crile stated, "palpable glands may be inflammatory and impalpable glands may be carcinomatous." "A strict rule of excision should therefore be followed." He further recommended against handling of the malignant tissue due to the lymphatic channels remaining intact that would encourage dissemination of the malignancy. Finally, he indicated that a tracheostomy was "doubly indicated" since aside from the short-circuiting of respiration and fixing the trachea, it produced a wall of protective granulations across the top of the precarious mediastinal area that therefore forestalled dissemination of disease into the chest.

Early in the introduction of his 1906 paper, Crile astutely identified that the immediate extension from the primary malignant focus principally occurred by permeation and metastasis in the regional lymphatics. As such, Crile summarized his recommendations for surgical management of the neck by stating that an incomplete operation would lead to dissemination of disease, stimulate the growth of the cancer, shorten the patient's life, and diminish comfort. He re-emphasized his philosophy that isolated excision of the primary focus of the cancer was "as unsurgical as excision of a breast" in the case where the regional lymph nodes remained unaddressed. Further, he offered support of en bloc removal of cervical lymph nodes in that excision of individual lymphatic glands would not result in cure of the patient, but it would rather be followed by greater dissemination and more rapid growth. He emphasized that a block dissection of the regional lymphatics and the primary malignancy was necessary, therefore, for effective treatment of these patients. This block dissection included lymph nodes in levels I–V of the neck (Table 1.1), the sternocleidomastoid muscle, the internal jugular vein, and the spinal accessory nerve. Crile performed this treatment in the management of patients in whom lymph nodes were enlarged (cN+ neck) as well as in those patients whose lymph nodes

Table 1.1 Oncologic levels of cervical lymph nodes

Cervical lymph node level	Location and anatomic boundaries
IA (submental)	Lymph nodes within the triangular boundary of the anterior belly of the digastric muscles and the hyoid bone
IB (submandibular)	Lymph nodes within the boundaries of the anterior belly of the digastric muscle and the stylohyoid muscle and the inferior border of the mandible
IIA and IIB (upper jugular)	Lymph nodes located around the upper third of the internal jugular vein and the adjacent spinal accessory nerve. Level IIA lymph nodes are located anterior (medial) to the spinal accessory nerve. Level IIB lymph nodes are located posterior (lateral) to the spinal accessory nerve
III (middle jugular)	Lymph nodes located around the middle third of the internal jugular vein. These nodes are located between the inferior border of the hyoid bone and the inferior border of the cricoid cartilage
IV (lower jugular)	Lymph nodes located around the lower third of the internal jugular vein. These nodes extend from the inferior border of the cricoid cartilage to the clavicle
V (posterior triangle)	Lymph nodes located along the lower half of the spinal accessory nerve and the transverse cervical artery. The supraclavicular nodes are located in this group of lymph nodes
VI (central compartment)	Lymph nodes in the prelaryngeal, pretracheal, paratracheal, and tracheoesophageal groove. The boundaries are the hyoid bone to the suprasternal notch and between the medial borders of the carotid sheaths. These lymph nodes are generally not dissected in oral cancer patients
VII (superior mediastinal)	Lymph nodes in the anterior superior mediastinum and tracheoesophageal grooves, extending from the suprasternal notch to the innominate artery. These lymph nodes are generally not dissected in oral cancer patients

were not clinically enlarged (cN0 neck). Crile's comments were collectively directed to head and neck cancer of a variety of anatomic sites. In his 1906 discussion, oral cavity cancers represented only a minority, including four cases of floor of mouth cancer, two alveolar ridge cancers, and 12 cancers of the tongue. Four cases of oropharyngeal cancer were reported including two cases of tonsillar cancer and one case each of soft palate cancer and pharyngeal cancer. This notwithstanding, this paper served as a model for treatment of the neck in patients with oral cancer. Interestingly, the most common cancer treated by Crile in his report of 132 cancers was that of the lips, accounting for 31 of these cases. By twenty-first century standards, most of these lip cancers could likely have been managed without neck dissection. There were no deaths related to these 31 lip cancers. Moreover, while the frequently quoted theme of Crile's paper was radical neck dissection, only 36 patients underwent such treatment in his report. Ninety-six patients reportedly did not undergo "radical block dissection."

In his 1923 paper [16] entitled *Carcinoma of the jaws, tongue, cheek, and lips*, Crile elaborated on his recommendations for excision of the cervical lymph nodes. He emphasized that early cancer of the gingiva or cheek that metastasizes late does not demand excision of the lymph nodes, while cancer of the lip, however early, demands the complete excision of all lymph nodes that drain the involved area. Further, cancer of the tongue or of the lip calls for the complete removal of the lymph nodes of the neck on both sides [16]. Crile's 1923 paper reiterated many of the statements made in the 1905 and 1906 papers, including comments about a review of 4500 reported autopsies of patients with head and neck cancer in which only 1% identified distant metastases. He emphasized that when death results from a cancer of the head and neck that local and regional disease was responsible for death rather than distant disease.

Dr. Crile's three papers represented the landmark articles regarding neck dissections for head and neck cancer until Dr. Hayes Martin published his paper entitled *Neck dissection* [17] in 1951. This extensive review commented on an experience of 1450 neck dissections performed from 1928 to 1950, although statistics were derived from 665 operations performed in 599 patients. One hundred forty-four patients with tongue cancer constituted the most common primary site, and these patients underwent 131 unilateral neck dissections and 13 bilateral neck dissections. Dr. Martin did not believe that a routine prophylactic radical neck dissection (RND) was practical in managing patients with cancer of the tongue and lip and presented data from a survey sent to 75 of his colleagues, the consensus of which supported his contentions. His conclusion regarding the RND was that routine prophylactic neck dissection was considered "illogical and unacceptable" for cancer of the oral cavity. He made these comments, due to his thoughts about oncologic safety and not about functional consequences, stating that no one could carry out prophylactic neck dissection to a degree sufficient to effect significant improvements in cure rates. He believed that the RND was an excessively radical technique performed electively and routinely. Stated differently, the RND should not be employed for the N0 neck, a philosophy that is largely observed in the twenty-first century. Regarding the elective neck dissection, Martin reported that this concept was not performed on the Head and Neck Service of Memorial Hospital at the time. Rather, he believed that definite clinical evidence that cancer was present in the lymph nodes represented one criterion for neck dissection. Other criteria included the requirement of control of the primary lesion giving rise to the metastasis, or if not controlled, there should be a plan to remove the primary cancer simultaneously with the neck dissection. Moreover, Martin indicated that there should be a reasonable chance of complete removal of the cervical metastatic cancer, there should be no clinical or radiographic evidence of distant metastasis, and the neck dissection should offer a greater chance of cure than radiation therapy.

While the RND has proved to be a reliable method of treating patients with oral/head and neck cancer, it is associated with substantial morbidity. Nahum [18] described a syndrome of pain and decreased range of abduction in the shoulder following RND. These symptoms constitute shoulder syndrome and relate to the sacrifice of the spinal accessory nerve (SAN). Preservation of the SAN during neck dissection ameliorates the syndrome [19]. The morbidity of the RND, therefore, gave way to the development of the numerous modifications of the RND that maintain oncologic safety while also reducing morbidity of the RND. These modifications of the RND were designed to preserve one or more of the sternocleidomastoid muscle, spinal accessory nerve, and internal jugular vein and have been realized in the form of the modified radical neck dissection (MRND) proper, and the selective neck dissections were represented primarily by the supraomohyoid neck dissection and secondarily by the functional neck dissection. By twenty-first century standards, radical and MRNDs are most commonly performed as *therapeutic* neck dissections for clinically N+ disease, while selective neck dissections are most commonly performed as *elective* neck dissections for clinically N0 disease.

Cervical Lymph Nodes in Relation to Oral Cancer and Classification of Neck Dissections

Surgical management of the cervical lymph nodes in patients with oral/head and neck squamous cell carcinoma requires a thorough understanding of the lymphatic anatomy of the neck and the patterns of nodal metastasis from these cancers. Classifications for neck dissections by the American Head and Neck Society [20, 21] reviewed six lymph node levels (Table 1.1) for defining the boundaries of neck dissection, levels I–V of which are potentially involved with oral squamous cell carcinoma (Fig. 1.1). In addition, lymph nodes in levels I–III are designated as sentinel, or first echelon lymph nodes for oral cavity cancers. Specifically, these are the first lymph nodes that will typically contain metastatic squamous cell carcinoma when the cervical lymph nodes in fact contain cancer. This well-accepted concept forms the basis for elective neck dissections where the likelihood of occult neck disease exceeds 20% [4].

Fig. 1.1 The oncologic lymph node levels of the neck as applied to oral cavity squamous cell carcinoma. (With permission from Regezi et al. [70])

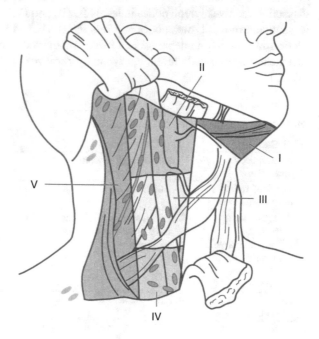

To develop uniformity regarding nomenclature, Robbins et al. [20] developed standardized neck dissection terminology in 1991 and updated the classification in 2002 [21] (Table 1.2). Their original classification was based on the following concepts: (1) the RND is the fundamental procedure to which all other neck dissections are compared, (2) MRND denotes preservation of one or more nonlymphatic structures, (3) selective neck dissections denote preservation of one or more group(s) of lymph nodes, and (4) extended RND denotes removal of one or more additional lymphatic and/or nonlymphatic structure(s). A modified radical neck dissection refers to the excision of all lymph nodes routinely removed by radical neck dissection with preservation of one or more nonlymphatic structures such as the spinal accessory nerve, internal jugular vein, and sternocleidomastoid muscle. Therein, lymph node levels I–V are removed in this neck dissection (Table 1.1). Typically, a type I MRND involves preservation of the spinal accessory nerve; a type II MRND involves preservation of the spinal accessory nerve and the internal jugular vein; and a type III MRND involves preservation of the spinal accessory nerve, internal jugular vein, and the sternocleidomastoid muscle [22]. It seems that most authors favor the type I MRND for the cN+ neck in oral/head and neck cancer [23] (Fig. 1.2), and this modification of the traditional RND does not compromise oncologic safety [24].

Neck dissections are additionally classified as *comprehensive* or *selective*. Comprehensive neck dissections are those where cervical lymph nodes are removed in levels I–V. Such neck dissections are represented by the radical and modified radical neck dissections for N+ disease, and commonly also remove nonlymphatic tissue. Selective neck dissections are those where cervical lymph nodes are selectively removed, and most commonly for cN0 disease. The most commonly performed selective neck dissection for oral cavity cancer is the supraomohyoid neck dissection that removes lymph nodes in levels I, II, and III. The anterolateral neck dissection removes lymph nodes in levels II, III, and IV, and the posterolateral neck dissection removes lymph nodes in levels II, III, IV, and V. The functional neck dissection is a poorly understood and often misquoted neck dissection in terms of sacrifice of lymph node levels but typically removes lymph nodes in levels II, III, IV, and V.

Table 1.2 Classification of neck dissections

1991 Classification	2001 Classification
1. Radical neck dissection	1. Radical neck dissection
2. Modified radical neck dissection	2. Modified radical neck dissection
3. Selective neck dissection (a) Supraomohyoid (b) Lateral (c) Posterolateral (d) Anterior	3. Selective neck dissection: each variation is depicted by "SND" and the use of parentheses to denote the levels or sublevels removed
4. Extended neck dissection	4. Extended neck dissection

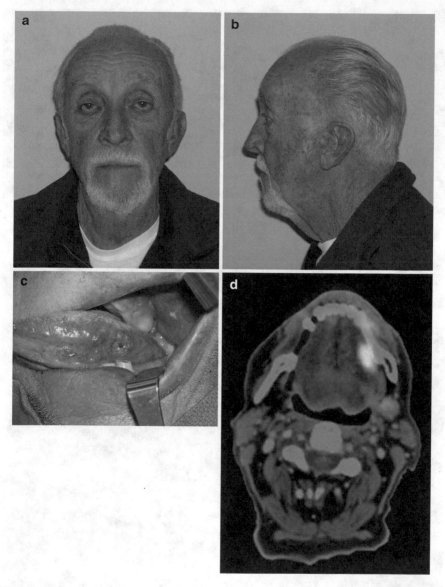

Fig. 1.2 A 71-year-old man (**a** and **b**) presented with a 2.5 cm area of mucosal ulceration and submucosal induration in the left tongue (**c**). Evaluation of the cervical lymph nodes identified a palpable 1.5 cm left level II mass. An incisional biopsy of the left tongue identified squamous cell carcinoma. Staging was consistent with a T2N1M0 cancer. PET/CT scans demonstrated hypermetabolic activity in the left tongue (**d**) and level II nodes of the left neck (**e** and **f**). Due to the patient's cN+ designation, a type I modified radical neck dissection was planned. A Crile incision was designed (**g**) and the MRND neck dissection specimen is noted (**h** and **i**). The resultant defect in the neck is appreciated (**j**). The patient simultaneously underwent left partial glossectomy with 1.5 cm margins (**k**). Three of 41 lymph nodes contained metastatic squamous cell carcinoma on microscopic examination. The tongue specimen demonstrated perineural invasion. The patient underwent postoperative radiation therapy and demonstrated no evidence of disease at 3 years postoperatively (**l**, **m**, and **n**)

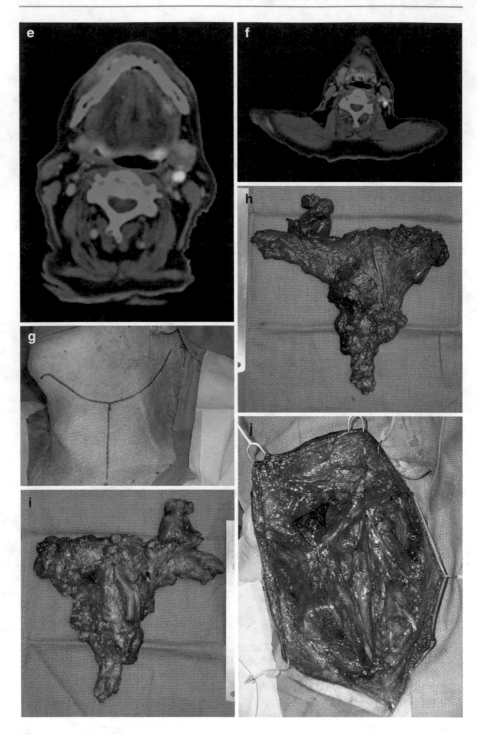

Fig. 1.2 (continued)

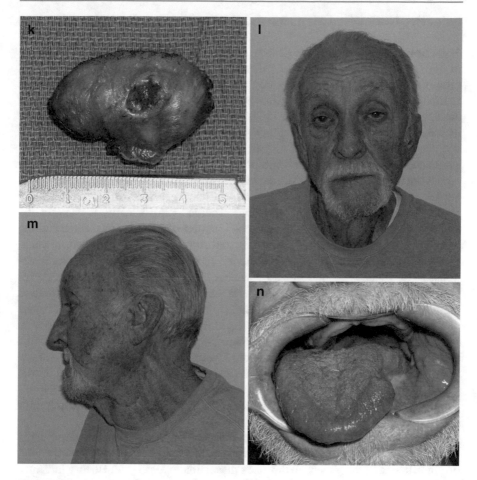

Fig. 1.2 (continued)

Comprehensive Neck Dissections for the Clinically Positive Neck

Type I Modified Radical Neck Dissection

The surgical concepts of modified radical neck dissections (MRNDs) are based on the understanding that the aponeurotic system of the neck encases the internal structures that are usually removed during RND. The MRND works within these planes of dissection and still results in an en bloc lymphadenectomy while preserving structures including the spinal accessory nerve, the sternocleidomastoid muscle, and the internal jugular vein. By definition, the type I modified radical neck dissection sacrifices lymph node levels I–V, the sternocleidomastoid muscle, and underlying internal jugular vein while intentionally preserving the spinal accessory nerve (Fig. 1.2). Most head and neck cancer surgeons preferentially execute this neck dissection for surgical management of the cN+ neck.

Selective Neck Dissections for the Clinically Negative Neck

Functional Neck Dissection (II–V)

In 1967, Bocca and Pignataro published their work on a more conservative neck dissection [25] that has been referred to as the functional neck dissection (FND). Lymph nodes in levels II–V are removed with intentionality in this selective neck dissection. Bocca and Pignataro indicated, "if the submaxillary fossa must be included in the dissection, the sacrifice of the submaxillary gland can generally be avoided because the gland itself may be easily stripped of its aponeurotic sheath." These authors also reported the flexibility of inclusion of a level I dissection in this procedure in 1980, indicating "the superficial cervical fascia is cut along the lower border of the submaxillary fossa against the lateral surface of the submaxillary gland, preserving the marginal mandibular nerve" [26]. Clearly, it was not the author's intention to execute a complete dissection of level I structures including lymph nodes in this region [27]. Feldman and Applebaum [28] provided justification for the exclusion of level I lymph nodes in their evaluation of 51 neck dissections, 26 of which were performed for cancer of the larynx and 12 of which were performed for cancer of the oral cavity. The results of their study identified three of the 51 neck dissections containing metastatic disease in level I of the neck. Of those three cases with metastatic level I disease, one specimen was a stage II floor of mouth cancer and one specimen was a stage IV retromolar cancer. None of the 12 laryngeal cancers demonstrated metastatic level I disease. By twenty-first century standards, ablative surgeons cannot equate the lymph node drainage patterns of oral cancer and laryngeal cancer such that a functional neck dissection, while scientifically justified for the treatment of laryngeal cancer, cannot be similarly justified for the treatment of oral cancer.

The first author to describe the functional neck dissection was Osvaldo Suarez from the University of Cordoba Medical School in Argentina. He published the first, original, systematic approach to this neck dissection in 1963 [15]. History indicates that Bocca learned the technique from Suarez and later published numerous observations on this technique as an elective neck dissection. Prior to that time, the elective neck dissection was the RND. In their report, the authors described absence of lymphatic recurrences in about 100 neck dissections where only the lymphatic tissue of the neck was sacrificed and the sternocleidomastoid muscle, internal jugular vein, and spinal accessory nerve were preserved. In 1984, these authors published their findings of 1500 functional neck dissections in 843 patients operated between 1961 and 1982 [29]. Cancer of the larynx comprised 87% of the patients in this series. Twelve hundred of these neck dissections were elective (cN0), while 300 were therapeutic (cN+). Neck recurrences occurred in 68 cases (8.1%). Of these, 16 occurred in the elective FND patients (2.38%) for N0 disease, and 52 recurrences occurred in the 171 therapeutic FND patients (30.4%) for N+ disease. Calearo and Teatini reviewed 476 functional neck dissections that were performed in 211 patients with only nine recurrences (3.5%) during a 3-year follow-up period [30]. Other authors [31, 32] have expressed similar satisfaction with this neck dissection.

Supraomohyoid Neck Dissection (I–III)

The supraomohyoid neck dissection is the ideal solution to the dilemma for some surgeons as to how to properly manage the cN0 neck associated with oral cavity cancer [33] (Fig. 1.3). A significant body of literature supports the performance of

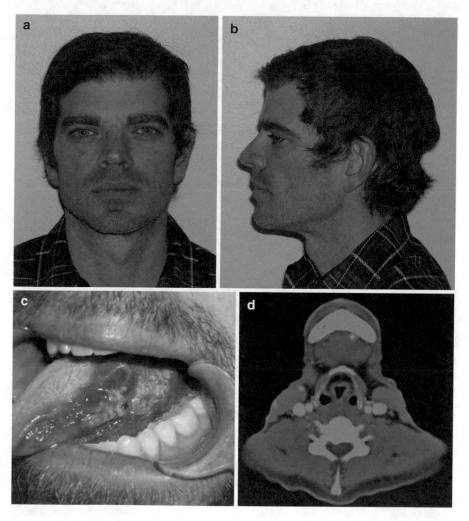

Fig. 1.3 A 37-year-old man (**a** and **b**) with a 5-cm left tongue mass (**c**) that was tender to palpation. An incisional biopsy was performed that identified squamous cell carcinoma. Staging was consistent with a T3N0M0 cancer. A PET/CT (**d**) was obtained that did not identify hypermetabolic activity associated with the cervical lymph nodes. The patient underwent a left supraomohyoid neck dissection (**e** and **f**) with identification and preservation of branches of the external carotid artery and internal jugular vein (**g**). A left hemi-glossectomy with 1 cm linear margins was performed (**h**, **i**, and **j**) and reconstructed with a radial forearm free microvascular flap (**k**). The patient's final pathology identified 1/20 lymph nodes with metastatic squamous cell carcinoma and perineural invasion in the tongue specimen. He underwent postoperative radiation therapy and remains free of disease at 4 years postoperatively (**l**, **m**, and **n**)

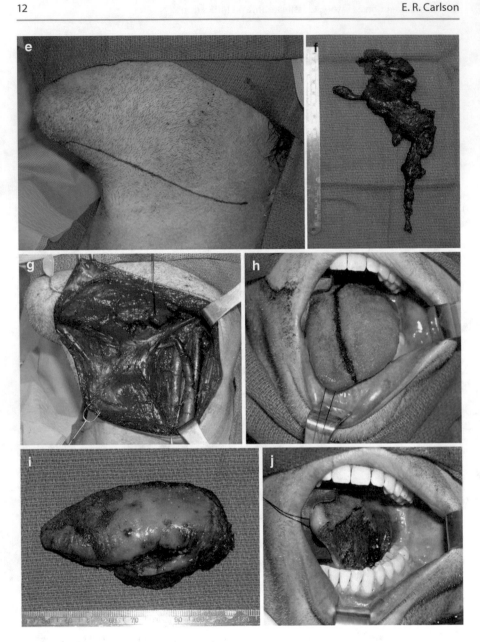

Fig. 1.3 (continued)

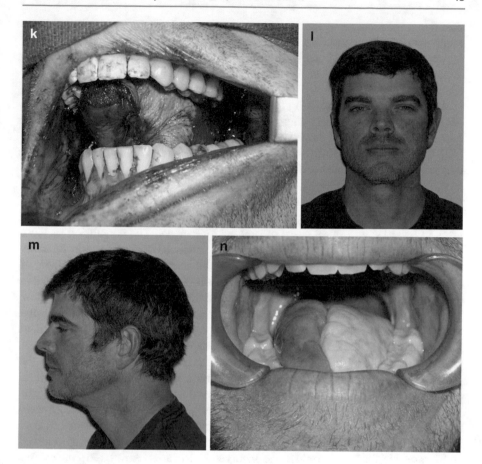

Fig. 1.3 (continued)

elective neck dissections for T1N0 and T2N0 squamous cell carcinomas of the oral cavity, identifying the incidence of occult neck disease in these cases of 36–42% [34–36]. As such, numerous authors have enthusiastically recommended the supra-omohyoid neck dissection as a staging procedure in the management of the N0 neck associated with oral cavity squamous cell carcinoma [37–41].

The supraomohyoid neck dissection removes lymph node levels I–III while pre-serving the spinal accessory nerve, internal jugular vein, and sternocleidomastoid muscle. This author shares the opinion of many others that delaying elective surgery of the cN0 neck and adopting the watchful approach to the cN0 neck is deleterious in most cases. This is particularly true for tongue cancer where survival in the watchful waiting group has been noted to be 33% compared to 55% in the neck dis-section group, and that locoregional control increased from 50% to 91% when neck dissection was performed [42]. The supraomohyoid neck dissection is a straightfor-ward surgical procedure that requires little time to perform and offers prognostically significant information to the patient, as well as to the radiation oncologist who might otherwise be unable to render treatment based on objective information. Most importantly, it addresses neck disease in an occult stage whereby survival is improved [8]. Its scientific basis is the observation that lymph nodes in levels I–III are sentinel nodes.

In a study by Shah examining the specimens of 501 patients undergoing radical neck dissection, only 9% of patients showed histopathological evidence of cervical lymph node metastases in level IV when the neck dissection was *elective* in nature [43]. The incidence of positive nodes in level V was only 2%. These data indicate that levels IV and V probably do not require removal in the management of the cN0 neck. This notwithstanding, Shah [44] recommended the excision of level IV lymph nodes along with levels I, II, and III when operating the cN0 neck related to primary cancers of the lateral border of the oral tongue. Crean et al. [45] found occult metastases in level IV in 5 of 49 cases of oral cavity cancers. The conclusion of these authors was that extending the traditionally performed SOHND to include the easily accessible level IV should be adopted as standard treatment in the management of the cN0 neck. Byers et al. [46] identified an overall frequency of skip metastases in squamous cell carcinoma of the oral tongue in 15.8% of their patients studied. These patients either demonstrated level IV metastases as the only manifestation of disease in the neck or the level III node was the only positive node present without disease in level I and II. The authors' conclusions were that the usual supraomohyoid neck dissection is inadequate for a complete pathologic evaluation of all the nodes at risk for patients with squamous carcinoma of the oral tongue. Feng et al. [47] retrospectively studied 637 patients with oral squamous cell carcinoma, particularly regarding skip metastases at level IV or V. Clinically negative necks were identified in 447 patients. The highest rate of occult metastasis was located at level II in these 447 patients, accounting for 74 cases (16.6%), while level I was involved in 67 cases (15.0%), and level III was involved in 16 cases (3.6%). Skip metastases were identified in 5 of the 447 cN0 patients (1.1%). No skip metastasis to level IV alone was observed in this study. The authors concluded that the supraomohyoid neck dissection is the preferred neck dissection in cN0 patients with oral squamous cell carcinoma.

Some authors have recommended performing the supraomohyoid neck dissection with frozen section analysis of the lymph nodes to permit intraoperative extension of the neck dissection in the form of a modified radical neck dissection [48, 49]. Other authors have stressed the importance of including level IV beyond the traditional supraomohyoid neck dissection when managing the cN0 neck where the primary tumor is located in the tongue [46, 50]. While many surgeons do not advocate the use of the supraomohyoid neck dissection in the management of the N+ neck, some recent evidence suggests the efficacy of this type of neck dissection with postoperative radiation therapy in the management of head and neck cancer patients with a cN+ neck [51]. This approach remains controversial and not oncologically safe if extracapsular extension of metastatic cervical lymph node disease is diagnosed microscopically. The supraomohyoid neck dissection is therefore not recommended by this author for the management of the cN+ neck.

Indications for Neck Dissection and Their Outcomes

This author performs surgical treatment of the neck primarily utilizing two main neck dissections. In patients with a clinically N0 neck, the sentinel or first echelon nodes are present in levels I, II, and III. As such, a supraomohyoid neck dissection as described would adequately address the neck in these patients (Fig. 1.3). As discussed, stage I and II squamous cell carcinoma of the tongue is a disease with a threshold incidence of occult neck disease thereby warranting elective treatment of the neck. This author does not adopt the wait-and-watch approach in such circumstances. The use of the supraomohyoid neck dissection in patients who have pathologically negative nodes has resulted in excellent control of disease in the neck with failure rates of less than 10% [43]. In the 30% of patients who are found to have pathologically proved occult neck disease, the failure rate with the supraomohyoid neck dissection alone ranges from 10% to 24% depending on the number of positive nodes and the presence of extracapsular spread [52]. When postoperative radiation therapy is added to this scenario, the failure rates drop to 0–15%, again depending on the extent of nodal metastases [53].

In patients with palpable cervical metastasis (N+), the levels at highest risk are levels I–IV. In the opinion and experience of this author, the most prudent operation to perform is the type I modified radical neck dissection, thereby sparing the spinal accessory nerve provided it is not involved with tumor (Fig. 1.2). This approach is recommended since palpable nodes smaller than 3 cm in diameter have a substantial incidence of extracapsular spread of disease [54]. The presence of extracapsular spread may breech the aponeurotic planes relied upon when the SCM and IJV are otherwise preserved. As such, a selective neck dissection is probably contraindicated in managing the cN+ neck related to oral cavity cancer [52]. In patients with clinically palpable neck disease, the results of type I MRND followed by postoperative radiation therapy depend upon the bulk of disease in the neck, the presence of extracapsular spread in the lymph node, and the radiosensitivity of microscopic disease remaining in the neck. When patients receive radiation therapy following a type I MRND for an N+ neck, neck failure rates in N1 patients are 7–10% and approximately 12% in N2 patients [55]. These results compare favorably to those obtained with RND in similar patients [52]. It is therefore oncologically safe and appropriate to preserve cranial nerve XI as part of a modified radical neck dissection.

While a great deal of thought must be exerted in determining which neck dissection is best suited for patients with oral cancer, perhaps the more controversial aspect of oral cancer care surrounds the small cohort of patients who *do not* require a neck dissection for effective management of their oral cancer. Due to the relative lack of morbidity and high yield of the supraomohyoid neck dissection in managing the cN0 neck, it seems reasonable to perform this neck dissection in most, if not all patients with squamous cell carcinoma of the oral cavity. This notwithstanding, there are some patients with early oral cancer for whom elective neck dissection is not necessary. In general terms, this author believes that the risk of occult neck disease is less than 20% in some patients with primary T1N0 and T2N0 cancers of the lip and anterior maxillary and anterior mandibular gingiva squamous cell carcinoma. As such, elective neck dissections may not be required in these patients in specific clinical circumstances. Robbins and Samant [56] indicate that a supraomohyoid neck dissection should be performed for all T1–T4 tongue cancers, T2–T4 at all other sites, and where there is identified perineural or lymphatic invasion in the primary specimen. Zhan et al. [57] analyzed 2,623 cases of primary cT1N0 squamous cell carcinoma in the National Cancer Database from 1998 to 2012, all of which underwent surgical resection and elective neck dissection. Most patients in the cohort were white (93%), men (60%), and operated at an academic medical center (58%). Forty-two percent of the cancers were primarily located in the oral tongue. Concordance with clinical and pathologic stage I designations occurred in 86% of cases. Occult nodal disease was 15% in this cohort. The incidence of occult nodal disease was higher in women (16.7%) than in men (13.9%; $P = 0.049$), and in moderately differentiated (17.4%) and poorly differentiated tumors (28.5%) than well-differentiated disease (5.9%; $P < 0.001$). Incidence did not vary significantly by age groups, race, academic versus community hospital, insurance type, or medical comorbidity. The authors concluded that elective neck dissection should be performed for moderately differentiated or poorly differentiated cT1N0 squamous cell carcinoma of the oral cavity, regardless of depth of invasion, and especially in women with tongue cancer. They also indicated that sentinel lymph node biopsy might represent a viable alternative for high-risk patients.

Brockoff et al. [58] investigated the threshold tumor depth of invasion of oral squamous cell carcinoma that would predict a 20% or greater risk of cervical lymph node metastases. The authors analyzed 286 patients in their database from 2009 to 2014. Most patients (94%) were white and the most common primary tumor site was the oral tongue (37%). The authors performed 390 neck dissections for these 286 patients, and 115 patients (40%) demonstrated cervical lymph node metastases. At 1-mm depth of invasion, the authors determined that none of the seven neck dissections demonstrated a positive node. At the 2-mm depth of invasion, there were 12 patients with node negative necks and 3 patients with node positive necks for an overall percentage of 20%. An increasing depth of invasion of greater than 2 mm resulted in a greater than 20% node positivity. The authors determined that the depth of invasion required for a 20% positivity rate of cervical lymph node metastases was 2 mm for tongue, 3 mm for floor of mouth, 3 mm for retromolar trigone, and 4 mm for alveolus/hard palate. The authors concluded that depth of invasion is an important factor to consider when establishing surgical recommendations for patients with T1N0 disease. This notwithstanding, the ultimate decision should be based on both the depth of invasion and the anatomic site of the primary tumor.

Kuo et al. [59] established guidelines for lymph node yield in patients with oral cavity squamous cell carcinoma while indicating that quality metrics were established for lymph node yield in regional node dissections for bladder, colorectal, esophageal, penile, and skin cancers. The authors analyzed 13,143 eligible cases of oral cavity cancer in the National Cancer Database. Patient factors that predicted a higher lymph node yield were male gender, young age, and African American race status. Of the patients who had known clinical lymph node staging ($n = 6147$), 71.1% underwent neck dissection. Most patients (79%) had cN0 disease, and the rate of neck dissection was 63.9% in these patients and 98.3% of cN+ patients underwent neck dissection. The lymph node yield was 21 lymph nodes overall, with 20 lymph nodes in the cN0 group and 25 lymph nodes in the cN+ group. Patients had significantly decreased survival when fewer than 16 lymph nodes were present in the neck dissections for cN0 patients and fewer than 26 lymph nodes in the neck dissections for cN+ patients.

The next genre of neck dissection is designated the *superselective neck dissection* utilizing sentinel node biopsies [60]. This technique was first described in melanoma patients [61], and it analyzes lymphoscintigraphy-guided biopsies of sentinel nodes in the neck to determine the histologic status of first echelon cervical lymph nodes and whether a neck dissection is indicated. Careful examination of a specific lymph node, as occurs in the evaluation of sentinel lymph node biopsies, but not elective neck dissections, may increase the utility of sentinel lymph node mapping. Ambrosch analyzed a series of 76 neck dissection specimens from patients originally staged as histologically negative [62]. The authors utilized ten-micron serial sections and hematoxylin-eosin staining and cytokeratin staining to re-assess the lymph nodes previously reported as negative. Eight previously undiagnosed micrometastases were identified in 6 specimens from 6 patients resulting in upstaging. Another study revealed 36 of 96 (37%) pathologically negative elective neck dissection specimens to contain micrometastases upon serial resectioning [63]. Similar findings have been noted by other authors [64, 65]. The consensus conclusion is that elective neck dissections might be therapeutic in a larger number of cases than previously thought. Serial sectioning is therefore essential in the processing of a sentinel lymph node [60].

In a study investigating the accuracy of sentinel lymph node biopsies in patients with squamous cell carcinoma, Shoaib [66] identified sentinel lymph nodes in 36 of 40 necks (90%). In four necks, nonsentinel lymph nodes contained tumor in the presence of pathologically positive sentinel lymph nodes. One case demonstrated a nonsentinel lymph node containing tumor, thereby giving the impression of a false-negative neck based on sentinel lymph node biopsies. Werner [67] reported that sentinel lymph node biopsies correctly identified metastatic disease in 97% of their 90 patients with head and neck squamous cell carcinoma. They indicated that if only the lymph node with the highest tracer activity was excised, 39% of cancer-positive necks would not be diagnosed. Payoux et al. [68] examined 30 patients with 37 neck dissections for N0 necks. Preoperative lymphoscintigraphy was performed and sentinel nodes were identified. In 29 necks, the sentinel node and neck dissection were negative for metastatic disease. Lymph node mapping allowed for identification of six of seven positive necks (86%). The authors concluded that lymphoscintigraphic sentinel node detection might have a role in the management of squamous cell carcinoma of the head and neck. The authors recommended that randomized clinical trials be performed before the technique is widely used.

Loree et al. [69] retrospectively analyzed the outcomes of sentinel lymph node biopsies in the management of previously untreated 108 patients with clinically negative necks related to oral squamous cell carcinoma. There were 56 T1, 49 T2, and two T3 tumors studied. The primary anatomic locations were 65 tongue, 7 floor of mouth, 13 buccal mucosa, 1 retromolar trigone, 15 lip, and 7 gingival cancers. The mean number of sentinel lymph nodes harvested per patient was two. Twenty-one patients (18.5%) had disease that was staged as SLN positive, and 82 patients (75.9%) had disease staged as SLN negative. The most common SLN site was ipsi-lateral level II (61 patients). Ten patients (9.7%) had their SLN identified outside of the boundaries of the supraomohyoid neck dissection. Sixteen patients (76%) with a positive SLN demonstrated lymph node metastases greater than or equal to 2 mm in size. Of these patients, five patients (31%) had additional nodal metastases on subsequent neck dissection. Of the 21 patients with positive SLN, all underwent selective or comprehensive neck dissection, six of whom demonstrated further posi-tive lymph nodes. Eight patients with positive SLN and either further positive lymph nodes, extracapsular extension or vascular invasion or perineural invasion at the primary site underwent chemoradiation therapy in the adjuvant setting. Of the 108 patients studied, 20 (19%) developed local, regional, or distant metastatic disease. Seven recurrences (6%) were nodal recurrences as false-negative SLN. The disease-specific survival (DSS) and disease-free survival (DFS) rates for the 108 patients were 93% and 81%, respectively. The DSS and DFS for patients with positive SNB were 91% and 76%, respectively. The authors concluded their study by indicating that sentinel lymph node biopsies may represent the superior modality for the man-agement of the cN0 neck in oral cavity squamous cell carcinoma.

Conclusion

Significant technical and philosophical refinement has occurred in neck dissections since 1905 in patients with oral/head and neck cancer. These refinements have been described and implemented in the best interests of enhancing the potential cure of these patients while also maintaining the patient's functional capacity and quality of life. One should anticipate that further developments will occur in this compelling surgical discipline in the future. In the meantime, ablative surgeons must strategi-cally execute surgical treatment for the clinically negative neck with the same degree of enthusiasm as is performed for the clinically positive neck, although clearly with different techniques.

References

1. Nahmias C, Carlson ER, Duncan L, et al. Positron emission tomography/computerized tomog-raphy (PET/CT) scanning for preoperative staging of patients with oral/head and neck cancer. J Oral Maxillofac Surg. 2007;65:2524–35.
2. Carlson ER, Schaefferkoetter J, Townsend D, et al. The use of multiple time point dynamic positron emission tomography/computed tomography in patients with oral/head and neck can-cer does not predictably identify metastatic cervical lymph nodes. J Oral Maxillofac Surg. 2013;71:162–77.
3. Schaefferkoetter JD, Carlson ER, Heidel RE. Can 3′-deoxy-3′-(^{18}F) fluorothymidine outper-form 2-deoxy-2-(^{18}F) fluoro-D-glucose positron emission tomography/computed tomography

in the diagnosis of cervical lymphadenopathy in patients with oral/head and neck cancer? J Oral Maxillofac Surg. 2015;73:1420–8.

4. Weiss MH, Harrison LB, Isaacs RS. Use of decision analysis in planning a management strategy for the stage N0 neck. Arch Otolaryngol Head Neck Surg. 1994;120:699–702.

5. Carlson ER, Cheung A, Smith BC, Pfohl C. Neck dissections for oral/head and neck cancer 1906–2006. J Oral Maxillofac Surg. 2006;64:4–11.

6. Carlson ER, Miller I. Management of the neck in oral cancer. Oral Maxillofac Surg Clin North Am. 2006;18:533–46.

7. Koyfman SA, Ismaila N, Crook D, et al. Management of the neck in squamous cell carcinoma of the oral cavity and oropharynx: ASCO clinical practice guideline. J Clin Oncol. 2019;37:1753–74.

8. D'Cruz AK, Vaish R, Kapre N. Elective versus therapeutic neck dissection in node-negative oral cancer. N Engl J Med. 2015;373:521–9.

9. Hamoir M, Holvoet E, Ambroise J, et al. Salvage surgery in recurrent head and neck squamous cell carcinoma: oncologic outcome and predictors of disease free survival. Oral Oncol. 2017;67:1–9.

10. Chung EJ, Park MW, Kwon KH, Rho YS. Clinical outcomes and prognostic factor analysis after salvage surgery for recurrent squamous cell carcinoma of the oral cavity. Int J Oral Maxillofac Surg 2020;49:285–91. September 4, Epub ahead of print.

11. Smith GI, O'Brien CJ, Clark J, Shannon KDF, Clifford AR, McNeil EB, et al. Management of the neck in patients with T1 and T2 cancer in the mouth. Br J Oral Maxillofac Surg. 2004;42:494–500.

12. Shah JP. Head and neck surgery in crisis. Preparing for the future (commentary). Arch Otolaryngol Head Neck Surg. 2005;113:556–60.

13. Crile G. Excision of cancer of the head and neck – with special reference to the plan of dissection based on one hundred and thirty-two operations. JAMA. 1906;47:1780–6.

14. Crile GW. On the surgical treatment of cancer of the head and neck. With a summary of one hundred and twenty-one operations performed upon one hundred and five patients. Trans South Surg Gynecol Assoc. 1905;17:108–27.

15. Ferlito A, Rinaldo A. Errare humanum est, in errore perseverare stultum: this is true also for neck dissection. Oral Oncol. 2005;41:132–4.

16. Crile GW. Carcinoma of the jaws, tongue, cheek, and lips. Surg Gynecol Obstet. 1923;36:159–62.

17. Martin H, Del Valle B, Ehrlich H, et al. Neck dissection. Cancer. 1951;4:441–99.

18. Nahum AM, Mullally W, Marmor L. A syndrome resulting from radical neck dissection. Arch Otolaryngol. 1961;74:82–6.

19. Short SO, Kaplan JN, Laramore GE, et al. Shoulder pain and function after neck dissection with or without preservation of the spinal accessory nerve. Am J Surg. 1984;148:478–84.

20. Robbins KT, Medina JE, Wolfe GT, Levine PA, Sessions RB, Pruet CW. Standardizing neck dissection terminology. Official report of the Academy's Committee for Head and Neck Surgery and Oncology. Arch Otolaryngol Head Neck Surg. 1991;117:601–5.

21. Robbins KT, Clayman G, Levine PA, Medina J, Sessions R, Shaha A, et al. Neck dissection classification update. Revisions proposed by the American Head and Neck Society and the American Academy of Otolaryngology – Head and Neck Surgery. Arch Otolaryngol Head Neck Surg. 2002;128:751–8.

22. Medina JE. A rational classification of neck dissections. Otolaryngol Head Neck Surg. 1989;100:169–76.

23. Myers EN, Fagan JJ. Treatment of the N+ neck in squamous cell carcinoma of the upper aerodigestive tract. Otolaryngol Clin North Am. 1998;31:671–86.

24. Khafif RA, Gelbfish GA, Asase DK. Modified radical neck dissection in cancer of the mouth, pharynx, and larynx. Head Neck. 1990;12:476–82.

25. Bocca E, Pignataro O. A conservation technique in radical neck dissection. Ann Otol Rhinol Laryngol. 1967;76:975–87.

26. Bocca E, Pignataro O, Sasaki CT. Functional neck dissection. A description of operative technique. Arch Otolaryngol. 1980;106:524–7.
27. Ferlito A, Rinaldo A, Robbins KT, et al. Changing concepts in the surgical management of the cervical node metastasis. Oral Oncol. 2003;39:429–35.
28. Feldman DE, Applebaum EL. The submandibular triangle in radical neck dissection. Arch Otolaryngol. 1977;103:705–6.
29. Bocca E, Pignataro O, Oldini C, et al. Functional neck dissection: an evaluation and review of 843 cases. Laryngoscope. 1984;94:942–5.
30. Calearo CV, Teatini G. Functional neck dissection. Anatomical grounds, surgical technique, clinical observations. Ann Otol Rhinol Laryngol. 1983;92:215–22.
31. Ariyan S. Functional radical neck dissection. Plast Reconstr Surg. 1980;65:768–76.
32. Gavilan J, Gavilan C, Herranz J. Functional neck dissection: three decades of controversy. Ann Otol Rhinol Laryngol. 1992;101:339–41.
33. Persky MS, Lagmay VMP. Treatment of the clinically negative neck in oral squamous cell carcinoma. Laryngoscope. 1999;109:1160–4.
34. Yuen APW, Lam KY, Chan CL, et al. Clinicopathological analysis of elective neck dissection for N0 neck of early oral tongue carcinoma. Am J Surg. 1999;177:90–2.
35. Ho CM, Lam KH, Wei WI. Occult lymph node metastasis in small oral tongue cancers. Head Neck. 1992;14:359–63.
36. Beenken SW, Krontiras H, Maddox WA. T1 and T2 squamous cell carcinoma of the oral tongue: prognostic factors and the role of elective lymph node dissection. Head Neck. 1999;21:124–30.
37. Henick DH, Silver CE, Heller KS, et al. Supraomohyoid neck dissection as a staging procedure for squamous cell carcinomas of the oral cavity and oropharynx. Head Neck. 1995;17:119–23.
38. Medina JE, Byers RM. Supraomohyoid neck dissection: rationale, indications, and surgical technique. Head Neck. 1989;11:111–22.
39. Kligerman J, Lima RA, Soares JR. Supraomohyoid neck dissection in the treatment of T1/T2 squamous cell carcinoma of oral cavity. Am J Surg. 1994;168:391–4.
40. Kowalski LP, Magrin J, Waksman G, et al. Supraomohyoid neck dissection in the treatment of head and neck tumors. Arch Otolaryngol Head Neck Surg. 1993;119:958–63.
41. Spiro JD, Spiro RH, Shah JP, et al. Critical assessment of supraomohyoid neck dissection. Am J Surg. 1988;156:286–9.
42. Jalisi S. Management of the clinically negative neck in early squamous cell carcinoma of the oral cavity. Otolaryngol Clin N Am. 2005;38:37–46.
43. Shah JP, Candela FC, Poddar AK. The patterns of cervical lymph node metastasis from squamous carcinoma of the oral cavity. Cancer. 1990;66:109–13.
44. Shah JP, Singh SG. Cervical lymph nodes. In: Head and neck surgery and oncology. 3rd ed. Edinburgh: Elsevier; 2003. p. 353–94.
45. Crean SJ, Joffman A, Potts J, Fardy MJ. Reduction of occult metastatic disease by extension of the supraomohyoid neck dissection to include level IV. Head Neck. 2003;25:758–62.
46. Byers RM, Weber RS, Andrews T, McGill D, Kare R, Wolf P. Frequency and therapeutic implications of "skip metastases" in the neck from squamous carcinoma of the oral tongue. Head Neck. 1997;19:14–9.
47. Feng Z, Li JN, Niu LX, Guo CB. Supraomohyoid neck dissection in the management of oral squamous cell carcinoma: special consideration for skip metastases at level IV or V. J Oral Maxillofac Surg. 2014;72:1203–11.
48. Manni JJ, van den Hoogen FJA. Supraomohyoid neck dissection with frozen section biopsy as a staging procedure in the clinically node-negative neck in carcinoma of the oral cavity. Am J Surg. 1991;162:373–6.
49. Van den Hoogen FJA, Manni JJ. Value of the supraomohyoid neck dissection with frozen section analysis as a staging procedure in the clinically negative neck in squamous cell carcinoma of the oral cavity. Eur Arch Otorhinolaryngol. 1992;249:144–8.
50. Woolgar JA. Pathology of the N0 neck. Br J Oral Maxillofac Surg. 1999;37:205–9.

51. Muzaffar K. Therapeutic selective neck dissection: a 25-year review. Laryngoscope. 2003;113:1460–5.
52. Shah JP, Andersen PE. Evolving role of modifications in neck dissection for oral squamous carcinoma. Br J Oral Maxillofac Surg. 1995;33:3–8.
53. Byers RM. Modified neck dissection. A study of 967 cases from 1970–1980. Am J Surg. 1985;150:414–21.
54. Snow GB, Annyas AA, Van Slooten EA, et al. Prognostic factors of neck node metastasis. Clin Otolaryngol. 1982;7:185–92.
55. Anderson PE, Spiro RH, Cambronero E, Shah JP. The role of comprehensive neck dissection with preservation of the spinal accessory nerve in the clinically positive neck. Am J Surg. 1994;168:499–502.
56. Robbins KT, Samant S. Neck dissection. In: Cummings CW, editor. Cummings otolaryngology head & neck surgery, Chapter 116. 4th ed. Philadelphia: Mosby; 2005. p. 2614–45.
57. Zhan KY, Morgan PF, Neskey DMP. Preoperative predictors of occult nodal disease in cT1N0 oral cavity squamous cell carcinoma: review of 2623 cases. Head Neck. 2018;40:1967–76.
58. Brockhoff HC, Kim RY, Braun TM, et al. Correlating the depth of invasion at specific anatomic locations with the risk for regional metastatic disease to lymph nodes in the neck for oral squamous cell carcinoma. Head Neck. 2017;39:974–9.
59. Kuo P, Mehra S, Sosa JA, et al. Proposing prognostic thresholds for lymph node yield in clinically lymph node-negative and lymph node-positive cancers of the oral cavity. Cancer. 2016;122:3624–31.
60. Myers EN, Gastman BR. Neck dissection: an operation in evolution. Arch Otolaryngol Head Neck Surg. 2003;129:14–25.
61. Morton DL, Wen D, Wong JH, Economou JS, Cagle LA, Storm FK, Foshag LJ, Cochran AJ. Technical details of intraoperative lymphatic mapping for early stage melanoma. Arch Surg. 1992;127:392–9.
62. Ambrosch P, Kron M, Pradler O, Steiner W. Efficacy of selective neck dissection: a review of 503 cases of elective and therapeutic treatment of the neck in squamous cell carcinoma of the upper aerodigestive tract. Otolaryngol Head Neck Surg. 2001;124:180–7.
63. Van den Brekel MWM, van der Wall I, Meijer CJLM, et al. The incidence of micrometastases in neck dissection specimens obtained from elective neck dissections. Laryngoscope. 1996;106:987–91.
64. Enepekides DJ, Sultanem K, Hguyen C. Occult cervical metastases: immunoperoxidase analysis of the pathologically negative neck. Otolaryngol Head Neck Surg. 1999;120:713–7.
65. Woolgar JA. Micrometastasis in oral/oropharyngeal squamous cell carcinoma: incidence, histopathological features and clinical implications. Br J Oral Maxillofac Surg. 1999;37:181–6.
66. Shoaib T, Soutar DS, MacDonald DG, et al. The accuracy of head and neck carcinoma sentinel lymph node biopsy in the clinically N0 neck. Cancer. 2001;91:2077–83.
67. Werner JA, Dunne AA, Ramaswamy A, et al. The sentinel node concept in head and neck cancer: solution for the controversies in the N0 neck? Head Neck. 2004;26:603–11.
68. Payoux P, Dekeister C, Lopez R, Lauwers F, Esquerre JP, Paoli JR. Effectiveness of lymphoscintigraphic sentinel node detection for cervical staging of patients with squamous cell carcinoma of the head and neck. J Oral Maxillofac Surg. 2005;63:1091–5.
69. Loree JT, Popat SR, Burke MS. Sentinel lymph node biopsy for management of the N0 neck in oral cavity squamous cell carcinoma. J Surg Oncol. 2019;120:101–8.
70. Regezi J, Sciubba J, Jordan RCK, editors. Oral pathology – clinical pathologic correlations, chapter 2. 7th ed. Philadelphia: WB Saunders Co.; 2017. p. 64. Figure 2-80

Complications Related to Skin Incisions, Design, and Skin Flaps

2

Waleed Zaid, Travis Williams, Rushil Dang, and Andrew Salama

Skin Anatomy and Physiology

It is essential to understand the anatomy of the skin, something that will lay a solid foundation to understand how tissues heal and offer an explanation as to why complications occur with neck dissection incisions and how to avoid them. Skin variations might include color, texture, thickness, and adnexal structure density. The adnexal structures include hair follicles, sebaceous glands, sweat glands, nerves, and blood vessels (Fig. 2.1).

Histological Layers of the Skin

The skin layer is classified into two distinct layers: the superficial epidermis and deeper dermis. The epidermis is composed of four sub-layers, including stratum basale, stratum spinosum, stratum granulosum, and stratum corneum. In terms of cells contained, the epidermis contains keratinocytes, melanocytes, Langerhans cells, and Merkel cells.

Langerhans cells are responsible for mediating skin's immune response and are found to be diminished in the skin of elderly patients and patients with chronic sun exposure, attributing to increased risk of skin cancers in this cohort of patients [1].

W. Zaid (✉) · T. Williams
Oral and Maxillofacial Surgery Department, Louisiana State University Health Sciences Center, New Orleans, LA, USA
e-mail: wzaid@lsuhsc.edu; twil60@lsuhsc.edu

R. Dang · A. Salama
Oral and Maxillofacial Surgery Department, Boston University – School of Dentistry, Boston, MA, USA
e-mail: Rushil.Dang@bmc.org; Andrew.Salama@bmc.org

© Springer Nature Switzerland AG 2021
T. Schlieve, W. Zaid (eds.), *Complications in Neck Dissection*,
https://doi.org/10.1007/978-3-030-62739-3_2

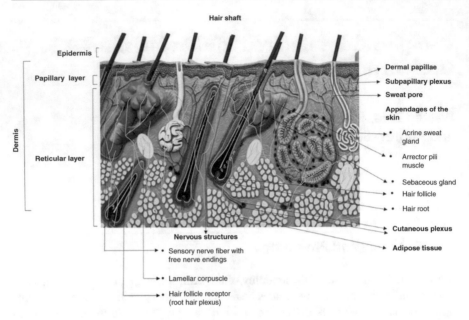

Fig. 2.1 Cross section of skin appendages, nerve supply, and blood supply. (Copied from Skin Anatomy and Morphology chapter from Skin Aging and Cancer, Springer)

Melanocytes are found in the basal layer and produce melanin, which protects keratinocytes from UV radiation and responsible for skin pigmentation. Darker pigmentation is not associated with an increased number of cells but more active melanocytes. Melanocyte concentration is notably diminished in elderly populations and, thus, may explain the increased risk of skin cancer in the elderly population [2]. The dermis consists of a thin superficial papillary and thick deep reticular layer. Dermal collagen fibers create its extensibility and strength, which decreases by 1% per year throughout adulthood [3]. Elastic fibers are responsible for the recoil and elastic properties of the skin. In solar-damaged skin, these fibers tend to bundle in the papillary dermis. Finally, the fibroblasts in the dermis are vital to wound healing because of the production of collagen, elastin, and ground substance. The fibrocyte may also become contractile during wound contraction [4–6].

Neurovascular Supply

Nerve supply includes sensory nerves responsible for pain, temperature, pressure, and proprioception. Autonomic nerves innervate blood vessels as well as appendage structures. The Merkel cell complex in the epidermis responds to touch, and Meissner corpuscles in the dermis mediate fine touch. The Pacinian corpuscles mediate deep pressure and vibration [4]. There are deep and superficial vascular plexuses that supply the blood flow to the skin. The deep vascular plexus is at the junction of subcutaneous fat and dermis. The superficial vascular plexus resides in the reticular dermis. Deep subcutaneous perforator vessels also exist in some regions of the face, including transverse facial, submental, and posterior auricular arteries [5].

Skin Physiology

General Skin Physiology

Thermoregulation and nutritional supply are both provided by the vascular system. Pre-capillary sphincters regulate the capillary supply of nutrition to the skin. These sphincters dilate during local hypoxemia leading to the accumulation of various metabolic by-products [6]. Thermoregulation is controlled by pre-arteriovenous shunt sphincters and the post-ganglionic sympathetic innervation. When the temperature is decreased, reduced norepinephrine is secreted compared to baseline leading to sphincter constriction. The blood supply is diverted from the skin due to the vasoconstriction; this results in decreasing temperature in the area with decreased blood supply. Adversely, when the body temperature is increased, more norepinephrine is secreted, causing vasodilation of the vessels to disperse heat and decrease the temperature [7]. The skin of the head and neck receives blood supply from 14 main arteries divided into two types, septocutanous and musculocutaneous arteries. Septocutaneous arteries pass directly within the fascia between muscles to the skin, and musculocutaneous pass through underlying muscles and have perforators that supply the overlying skin [5].

Skin Flap Design and Blood Supply

Most skin flaps performed in the head and neck region are random or axial flaps. Skin flap survival is interrelated with the length to width ratio [8]. Some authors believe that the flap viability is best related to the capillary perfusion pressure of a given area [4]. The perfusion pressure decreases as distance increases from the base to the distal flap. If this pressure drops low enough, the arterioles in the deep vascular plexus will constrict, causing ischemia and inevitably lead to necrosis of the skin flap. Therefore, making a flap wider may not improve survival if it does not increase perfusion pressure.

The Angiosome-Based Approach

Taylor and Palmer first described the angiosome concept in 1987, the concept describes multiple three-dimensional tissue blocks supplied by a particular source artery called angiosome, these angiosomes are connected via anastomotic vessels called "choke" vessels, their function is to regulate blood flow between the angiosomes. In the head and neck region, 13 angiosome territories have been defined with many angiosomes being irregular and convoluted. The primary vascular supply to the neck is from the subclavian, internal carotid, and external carotid systems [9, 10].

Implementing the angiosome concept to the skin and the subcutaneous tissues of the neck, it could be classified into four distinct areas:

1. The anterior midline neck supplied by the superior and inferior thyroid arteries
2. Upper lateral neck supplied by branches of the facial and occipital arteries
3. Mid lateral neck supplied again by the superior thyroid artery and deep cervical artery
4. Lower lateral neck supplied by the inferior thyroid and transverse cervical arteries

The dermal-subdermal plexus is continuous across the midline along with interconnections between the contralateral angiosomes [11].

Multiple overlapping angiosomes supply muscles in the neck, often consisting of a dominant principal source vessel and other less dominant vessels, and they can be grouped into three main groups:

1. Sternocleidomastoid: Dominantly supplied by the occipital and superior thyroid arteries. Other minor territories supplied by the inferior thyroid and transverse cervical arteries.
2. Scalene muscles, consisting of the scalenus anterior, scalenus medius, and scalenus posterior, which constitute the lateral group of muscles. The deep cervical artery supplies the inferior portion of the muscle bellies, and the ascending cervical artery supplies the superior portion.
3. Anterior neck muscles: The suprahyoid muscles are primarily supplied by the occipital; lingual and facial arteries and the infra-hyoid muscles are mostly supplied by the superior and inferior thyroid arteries.

With time, a thorough understanding of blood supply to the neck has led to several modifications in incision design, preventing skin necrosis, decreased wound breakdown, and improved aesthetic results.

Flap Tension

In the context of neck dissection, the survival of the developed skin flaps depends on the blood supply, which can be compromised with closure under tension. Upon initial stretching of the skin, a significant extension can occur with little effort. However, with increased stress on the skin, it becomes considerably more challenging to gain any movement of the skin flaps. Microscopically, the stretching of collagen and elastic fibers occur initially in the direction of applied force with little resistance of deformation. As additional force is applied, more collagen and elastic fibers are recruited. Eventually, all fibers are recruited and aligned in the direction of the force, and no further deformation is possible. With aged skin, there is a loss of elastic fibers, and their elastic recovery and less force are needed to achieve adequate skin mobilization (Fig. 2.2). This tends to result in less wound closure under tension with elderly patients. At maximal strain, there is no difference in skin tension in the elderly when compared to young patients. The number of collagen

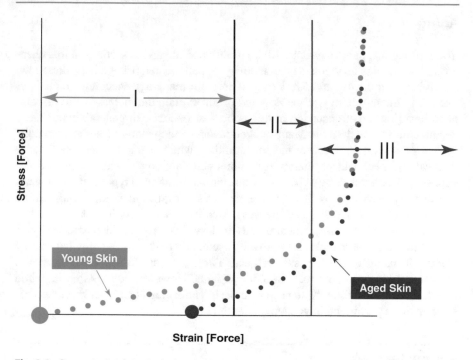

Fig. 2.2 Stress-strain curve for isolated skin

fibers decreases with age, not the elasticity. Using the stress-strain curve, flap necrosis is directly related to both the length of the flap and applied tension. At equal closing tensions, larger skin flaps will have a high possibility of necrosis.

Flap Undermining

Undermining skin flaps are rarely needed after a neck dissection; however, it might be required if there is a need to reconstruct small skin defects arising from the neck dissection. Undermining the flap will release vertical attachments between the dermis and underlying tissues. Consequently, the undermined flap can slide over the subcutaneous tissue. Surgeons must pay close attention to maintaining proper planes of dissection to maintain the feeding vessels to the skin flap; otherwise, this might lead to flap necrosis. Surgeons must be conscious of the extent of undermining performed compared to how much is required. Some studies show that >4 cm of undermining is unfruitful in reducing flap tension significantly and only increases the risk of flap necrosis. The increased flap necrosis rate may be because the perfusion pressure is not sufficient to supply the length of the flap [4].

Aging

You will see that the aging topic will be mentioned in various sections in this chapter and across this textbook, as the majority of patients requiring a neck dissection are in between the 4th and 5th decade. There are many age-specific skin changes that affect the physiology of the skin and might explain the increased rate of complications that might occurring in this cohort of patients. In general, aging has a negative impact on the skin. Many exogenous and endogenous causes can expedite aging of the skin; these causes include smoking, which is the most common cause of head and neck cancer, mainly squamous cell carcinoma, while excessive sun exposure a common cause of basal cell carcinoma. Epidermal regeneration capacity is adversely decreased by 50% in aged skin resulting in impaired wound healing [12]. With aging, skin collagen decreases in quality and quantity. The skin is thinned from collagen remodeling, which results in less elasticity but increased laxity. A benefit of increased wrinkles is improved ease of camouflaging the eventual scar by placing incisions at existing skin creases. There are data to support a decreased incidence of hypertrophic scars in older patients. However, due to often impaired and decreased blood supply, flaps in an elderly patient are at a higher risk of necrosis than those performed in younger patients [13].

Wound Healing

Wound healing is a stepwise cellular response that helps restore the structural and functional integrity of the skin. Head and neck cancer patients are known to have significantly increased risk of complications related to wound healing. Patients with advanced head and neck disease will need adjuvant therapy, ideally started within 6 weeks after surgical treatment, as recommended by the National Comprehensive Cancer Network [NCCN]. Optimizing wound healing is crucial in these patients to allow timely initiation of adjuvant therapy. Unfortunately only 44% of head and neck patients fall within that time frame, and "wound-healing issues" is one of the common reasons leading to delay in starting adjuvant therapy [14]. There are four stages of wound healing, and they include exudative, resorptive, proliferative, and maturation. Exudative involves hemostasis via platelet activation and scab formation.

The resorptive phase depends on cytokine release from macrophages to recruit other immune cells and fibroblasts. Recruited lymphocytes then promote cellular immunity and neutrophils, and macrophages will phagocytose pathogens and cellular debris. Granulation tissue develops during the proliferative phase. It involves macrophages, fibroblasts, and type III collagen. Epidermal stem cells proliferate to recreate new epidermis, and secretion of collagenase degrades the previously formed clot. Contraction occurs as collagen synthesis increases, and myofibroblasts pull the wound together. Finally, the remodeling phase replaces type III collagen with type I collagen. At this stage, the epidermis has finished forming without the regeneration of the follicles or cutaneous glands. The first initial stages take place within 2 weeks, but the final stage can continue for months. Many factors affect wound healing. They can be categorized into wound-related factors, such as wound size, tension, and location of the surgical wound, and systemic factors include medical comorbidities such as diabetes, peripheral vascular disease, and nutritional status. Malnutrition is common among head and neck cancer patients and has been linked to poor healing, as well as early mortality in this patient group [15]. Malnutrition is a fact that inspired various tumor boards to invite nutritionists to their multidisciplinary head and neck tumor boards [16]. The net result from compromised wound healing might result in a chronic wound and increased risk of surgical site infection simply due to the disruption of the functional skin barrier [17]. In the setting of neck dissections, wound-related complications tend to have a wide range between 3% and 34% [18]. Other factors include the surgeon's experience, patient compliance, and the dose of radiation therapy [18, 21]. Wound complications are higher in patients receiving radical or modified radical neck dissection than selective neck dissection [18]. Hypertrophic scars (Fig. 2.3) are related to increased collagen deposition, causing protrusion of the scar tissue from the surface of the skin that is confined within the original wound margins. Keloids, on the other hand, share increased collagen deposition with hypertrophic scars but also have additional fibroblast proliferation that expands beyond the original wound margins. In the setting of neck dissections, neck keloids are considered uncommon and occur more frequently in patients from African American or Asian backgrounds. Preoperative evaluation should include screening for a history of excessive scarring or keloid disorder. Patients with keloids tend to have family history of developing keloids or patients might report keloid formation from previous skin injuries or incisions [20].

Fig. 2.3 Hypertrophic scar 1-year post neck dissection

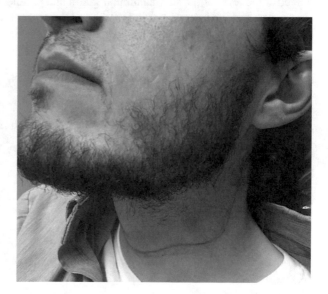

Skin Incision Designs

Surgical incision design is a critical portion of operative planning for neck dissection to allow adequate exposure to harvest a representable nodal yield and eliminate gross metastatic neck disease. The selection is often based on the surgeon preference and access required for optimum neck disease clearance without increasing the risk of complications and compromising vascularity. Incisions should be able to be closed with ease and directly avoid vital structures. Selection should also be based on other considerations such as laterality, neck disease location, the extent of the anticipated neck dissection, history of radiation or planned radiation, previous surgery, need for flap reconstruction, and finally if a concomitant tracheostomy is planned [19, 20]. Neck incision designs have been described in literature since the early 1900s with the landmark Y incision detailed in 1906 by Crile, who introduced the concept of radical neck dissection; this incision is less commonly used today [21]. As neck dissections became more popular and accepted, many incision designs were created. Physical characteristics such as neck flexibility, neck length, girth, muscle bulk, and fascial consistency are all factors, which may influence surgical incision planning. Patients with decreased neck extension, decreased thyromental distance, increased neck girth, and thick muscle bulk make the dissection more challenging, and these must be thoroughly evaluated in the preoperative visit.

MacFee Incision

The single transverse incision eventually gave rise to the MacFee incision (Fig. 2.4), which is composed of two horizontal parallel incisions: the superior incision is placed at the level of the submandibular gland and parallel to the mandible within a skin crease and the lower incision is placed at the supraclavicular area within a skin crease as well [22]. The main advantage of the MacFee incision is that it avoids any

Fig. 2.4 MacFee incision, the superior and inferior incisions are depicted with the straight black line; in the modified MacFee, the incisions are curved to reduce the distance between the two lines, depicted with the dotted lines

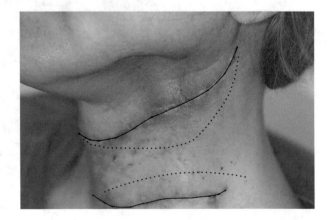

vertical incisions. MacFee incision might decrease exposure leading to the possibility of compromised disease clearance [23]. The two vertical extensions of the modified MacFee allow improved exposure while reducing the bridge between two horizontal incisions. The modified MacFee is less aesthetic than the original MacFee incision. On average, the MacFee incision takes longer to raise; this might be attributed to the distance between the two horizontal incisions and the strenuous task of tunneling between them [24]. MacFee himself reported on this, admitting that it was more difficult and time consuming than the vertical incision. Developing skin flaps arising from the MacFee incision may take longer to raise, but it is faster to close when compared with incisions. Closure time is improved because only two transverse skin incisions exist. The increased time to raise the flap is offset by the decreased closure time. The MacFee incision may not be suitable for patients with shorter neck length or less elastic neck skin. The posterior neck is also difficult to access with the MacFee [23, 24].

The Single Transverse Incision

Extending from anterior border of the trapezius muscle to the level of the cricoid cartilage, this incision is often used for thyroidectomy with a concomitant neck dissection. It provides good exposure and cosmesis, only if level I is not involved or not part of the desired dissected lymph nodes. The incision exposure might not be sufficient, especially in patients with long necks, high positive level II nodes, and in the need to explore level I [25, 26]. An adjusted transverse cervical incision might improve exposure of level I through V without extension. With this type of incision, the skin flap, the vasculature is random and is supplied from the platysma, and thus skin flaps should be raised in the subplatysmal plane. If a bilateral neck dissection is performed, it should not extend caudally to preserve the facial and occipital arteries for flap viability. This flap design should not be used if the platysma is adhered to underlying lymph nodes, or if the tumor has invaded the overlying skin. Some authors think this incision is superior to the MacFee as it requires less intensive retraction and decreases the risk of marginal ischemia [25, 26, 30]. The MacFee scar is not able to be concealed as well as the single transverse incision. Other incision designs such as the T and Y types also include tri-points, which are even more difficult to conceal and more likely to develop edge ischemia [31, 32]. There is less scarring with the transverse cervical incisions, while there was an increased risk of skin breakdown, especially those who underwent radiotherapy [26]. Ideally, incision design should provide some flexibility to the surgeon for intraoperative alterations or modification during the neck dissection procedure. Straight-line transcervical incisions are favored for this reason and their ability to provide safe, aesthetic, and rapid removal of the previously mentioned lymph node groups [19, 27]. The main advantage of the straight-line incision is that it can be placed in the cervical neck crease at a resting skin tension line, creating a barely perceptible scar. It relies on the elasticity of the skin and platysma. Therefore, it may not be appropriate in patients where skin elasticity is limited due to fibrosis or with extensive subcutaneous fat [28].

Schobinger Incision

Schobinger was the first to report a Y-type incision that placed the vertical component more posteriorly, rather than directly over the carotid (Fig. 2.5). It creates a long anterior- and posterior-based skin flaps, plus a superior flap [29]. This incision provides sufficient access to all five levels of lymph nodes and adequate exposure to the oral cavity (Fig. 2.6). This incision was slightly modified by adding a curve to the vertical component [22, 26].

The modified Schobinger's incision is one of the commonly used incisions for neck dissection, especially for bulky neck disease or if level V nodal group is involved [19]; however, the modified Schobinger incision has the worst scar formation compared to other incisions. The tripoint incision reduces blood supply to the tripartite point, causing ischemia and cosmetic compromise. Besides, the incision is

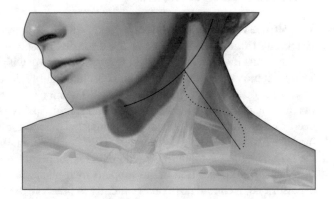

Fig. 2.5 Schobinger incision, the classical incision had a straight drop-down line, while the modification made that drop-down incision curvier "dotted line"

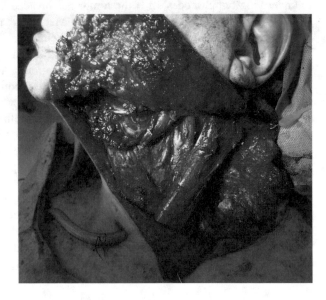

Fig. 2.6 Modified radical neck dissection [1-v], preserving the sternocleidomastoid [SCM] and the spinal accessory nerve

directed against the natural skin creases in a vertical direction, further creating an unacceptable scar [24, 30]. When the transverse cervical incisions were compared with Schobinger incision, the transverse cervical incisions demonstrated fewer cases of would infection and flap necrosis [26, 31]. Similarly, the Schobinger incision is more time consuming to raise due to the raising of anterior and posterior flaps [24].

The Apron Incision

The apron incision is the workhorse incision that provides almost equivalent exposure as the Tri-radiate, without its wound healing risks. Its main advantage is the extensive vascular supply arising from the external carotid to allow adequate healing even in the irradiated neck [32]. It is the author's preferred neck dissection incision, especially that it can be easily converted into a Schobinger or modified Schobinger. The other advantage of the apron incision is it can be incorporated with different approaches such as the lip-split approach (Fig. 2.7) or the modified Blair incision for parotid surgery (Fig. 2.8). The apron incision allows excellent neck dissection, and can be used to perform selective neck dissection, modified radical neck dissection, or even radical neck dissection in selected cases (Figs. 2.9 and 2.10).

Fig. 2.7 Apron incision incorporated with modified Blair parotid incision

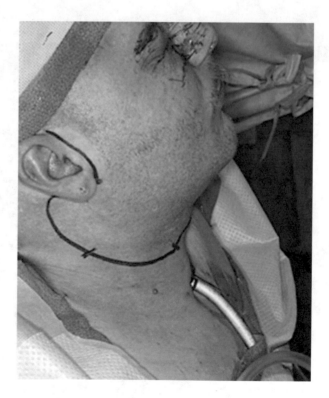

Fig. 2.8 Apron incision incorporated with a lip-split incision

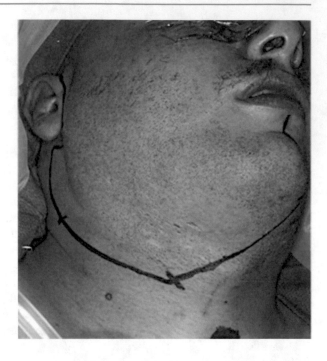

Fig. 2.9 Neck dissection bed after completion of a selective neck dissection [I-IV], performed via an apron incision

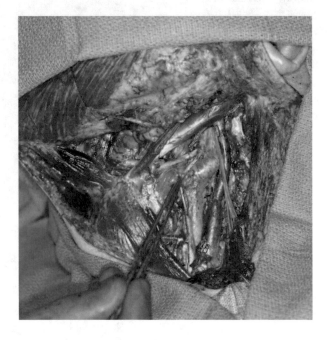

Fig. 2.10 Neck dissection bed after a radical neck dissection performed via an apron incision

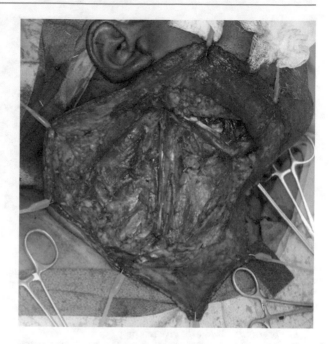

Risk Factors Related to Neck Dissection Skin Incisions

The most common complications associated with the skin incisions for neck dissections include delayed wound healing, which can lead to dehiscence. This consists of both deep and superficial dehiscence. Violation in the skin's natural protective barrier can then predispose those patients to surgical wound infections (Fig. 2.11).

Additionally, skin flap necrosis is another complication that occurs after a neck dissection and might compromise the vascular reconstruction if it was concomitantly performed. It is more common at the site of T intersections in skin incisions than single skin incisions. It can additionally occur if blood supply to skin flap is violated in case of excessive undermining or if the closure is performed under high tension. Finally, unaesthetic results are another complication of skin incision as no incision can be performed without minor scars. However, care should be taken to either prevent or reduce scarring as much as possible. Some systemic risk factors (Table 2.1) can place patients at a higher tendency for these aforementioned complications and should be noted and addressed in the preoperative planning stage. Studies have been performed demonstrating the risk of neck dissection on the previously treated neck, as patients with a history of prior surgery have increased scar tissue and altered anatomy that may impair wound healing and place the patient at increased risk for wound infection.

Additionally, many studies have found an increased risk of wound complications with a history of prior radiation/chemotherapy. As mentioned previously, nutrition is directly connected with proper wound healing, and thus those that are

Fig. 2.11 A case of [T4a, N2b, Mo] anterior mandibular gingival OSCC, that underwent composite segmantal manidbular resection, bilateral neck dissection and immediate reconstrcution with a fibula free flap, this patient developed skin necrosis and wound degiscence accrss the apron incision

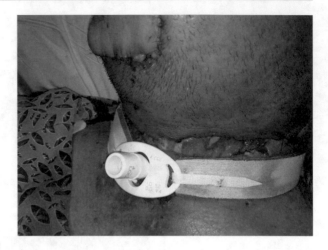

Table 2.1 Systemic risk factors for skin incision complications during a neck dissection

Risk factors for skin incision complications
Previously treated neck – surgery, radiation, chemotherapy
Poor nutritional status
History of keloids or excessive scarring
Past medical history that impairs wound healing – DM, PVD
Immunocompromised patients – HIV, Hep C, Hep B
Patients taking immunosuppressive medications [Ex. Solid organ transplant patients]

malnourished may be at increased risk of delayed wound healing. Additionally, patients with medical conditions like DM or PVD, and those with medical conditions that suppress the immune system can have a similar predilection for wound complications or skin flap necrosis. Finally, those with previous history of hypertrophic scarring or keloid formation are at increased risk of an unaesthetic result and excessive scarring.

Management of Skin Incision Complications

Prevention of Skin Incision Complications/General Considerations

The best way of managing complications of neck dissection is by minimizing them via preventive measures. This can be done through preoperative nutritional optimization, habit modification, medical optimization, and proper surgical planning and design of the skin incisions. A sound surgical technique is key to preventing complications. Local anesthesia use is optional; we prefer the use of local anesthesia as it helps to delineate dissection planes and assist with hemostasis. We also tend to use the backside of the blade to create hash marks that are marked with permanent ink to allow accurate re-approximation and closure of the skin at the end of the neck dissection procedure. We make skin incisions with electrocautery; other surgeons prefer the use of cold scalpel, our experience did not show any difference in wound infection and excessive scar formation, something that has been supported by published literature [33, 34]. Constant irrigation of the skin flaps and wrapping them with a moist lap or gauze is recommended (Fig. 2.12).

Nutritional Status/Diet Modification

Patients with head and neck cancer often present with malnutrition, oral cavity and oropharyngeal cancer patients may experience dysphagia or odynophagia providing inherent risk for poor PO intake and malnutrition, mechanical restriction as some of these patients suffer from severe trismus leading to decrease oral intake, alcohol abuse and during the adjuvant phase especially those patients undergoing chemotherapy, which can lead to nausea and vomiting. All these reasons might advocate for the preoperative placement of percutaneous gastrostomy tube to improve preoperative nutritional status and assistance with prompt feeding in the postoperative period; with that being said, we encourage patients to maintain oral intake even if a PEG tube was inserted [16]. Malnutrition directly correlates with delayed wound healing. Therefore, a nutritionist must be included as part of the head and neck cancer multidisciplinary team as it has been shown to improve outcomes. The patient's nutritional status should be assessed with screening tools during the initial evaluation and then repeated at intervals throughout treatment to ensure proper nutrition. Screening should be repeated weekly for inpatients, and weight should be recorded routinely at outpatient visits. Weight loss of 2 kg or more within 2 weeks should be reported to the nutritionist [41, 42]. Validated assessment tools include *scored Patient-Generated–Subjective Global Assessment* or *Subjective Global Assessment* [16]. Nutritional assessment parameters include clinical observation, diet history [recent intake], calculation of caloric requirements, and proposed treatment plan/intervention. Those with poor status should be referred to a dietary specialist and receive pretreatment intervention. Many long-standing lifestyle habits can negatively impact nutrition, such as smoking and alcohol dependence. Patients with unintentional weight loss greater than 10 percent in the preceding 6 months, place the patient at increased risk of infection, delayed wound healing, impaired

Fig. 2.12 Superiorly based skin flap elevated and secured with Lone star elastic self-retaining retractors after a wet surgical Lap is applied on the undersurface of the flap

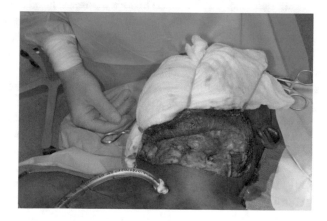

cardiorespiratory function, muscle weakness, depression, poor quality of life, postoperative complications, reduced response to chemoradiation therapy, and increased rate of mortality in head and neck cancer patients [16]. Therefore, early nutritional treatment for malnutrition should be initiated to improve clinical, self-reported patient symptoms, and financial outcomes. During preoperative clinical assessment, the surgeon should evaluate the patient's ability to chew and swallow and identify causes leading to weight loss and hints arising from weight loss [i.e., ill-fitting dentures/clothing]. The medical history should be reviewed concerning its effect on nutritional status, such as diabetes, Crohn's disease, or celiac disease. A BMI < 18 Kg/m^2 suggests malnutrition and should be addressed. Biochemical values are often easy to attain and can provide good insight into nutritional status. Overall, nutritional support aims to improve the subjective quality of life, enhance anti-tumor treatment effects, reduce adverse effects of anti-tumor therapies, and prevent and treat malnutrition. Nutritional support should be tailored to meet the needs of the patient and be realistic to achieve. There are three main methods of providing nutritional support: oral, enteral, and parenteral. Parenteral support is rarely used in head and neck cancer patients. Nutritional therapy, including protein optimization, holding caloric-restrictive diets, and food fortification should be initiated as soon as the decision of parenteral therapy is decided. If malnutrition already exists or is anticipated that the patient will be unable to eat for more than 7 days, enteral nutrition should be initiated. Inadequate intake occurs when 60% of estimated energy expenditure is unable to be consumed. If inadequate or minimal intake is anticipated for more than 10 days, standard polymeric feeds should be used. There should be a strong consideration for gastrostomy insertion if long-term feeding will be necessary for greater than 4 weeks. As energy requirements may change postoperatively, weight and intake should be monitored regularly to adjust intake as needed [19, 41].

Habit Modification

Social history is also a vital component of nutritional evaluation and should not be ignored. Patients should be questioned on alcohol intake, smoking, substance misuse, social support system, access to food or cooking skills, and social and financial circumstances. Support in overcoming these pitfalls can be provided to improve the overall outcome [16]. Tobacco history increases the risk of oral cancer and impairs wound healing postoperatively. A well-defined duration of smoking cessation that can reduce the risk of impaired wound healing is not present in the literature, but the earlier, the better. Conflicting results on smoking and wound healing postoperatively exist. Smoking cessation of 2 weeks before colorectal surgery did not reduce wound complications [35–37]. Another randomized control trial showed 4-week cessation of smoking led to decreased incisional wound infections [38]. Finally, a retrospective study of neck dissections demonstrated smoking cessation for 3 weeks or longer before surgery lowered the risk of impaired wound healing [35]. In general, patients suffering from smoking-related cancers have a high nicotine dependence, contributing to withdrawal symptoms such as agitation and disorientation [20]. Alcohol consumption among head and neck patients is also typical and leads to postoperative withdrawal symptoms and delirium tremens.

Medical Optimization

Delayed wound healing or chronic wounds occur most commonly in patients with systemic risk factors such as diabetes mellitus or peripheral vascular disease. Therefore, it is vital to ensure medical conditions are optimized prior to neck dissection surgery to reduce the risk of acute or chronic wound formation. Thus, patients prior to surgery should be sent to their primary care physician. If they do not have access to one, in an ideal world, these patients should be referred and establish care for medical optimization.

Surgical Planning/Technique

As demonstrated earlier in this chapter, a variety of incision designs exist, but the choice ultimately relies on the surgeon's preference and familiarity. The incisions for neck dissections should be placed to optimize blood flow. Trifurcation or incisions parallel to the carotid artery should be evaded, particularly in salvage cases after radiotherapy, as they have a higher rate of flap necrosis [39]. Increased risk of complications is associated with salvage neck dissection defined as a neck dissection that has been previously treated with surgery, chemotherapy, or radiation; this will be discussed in a separate chapter. However, salvage neck dissections have increased risk of dehiscence and skin flap necrosis, leading to a need for an increased hospital stay and additional surgery [40, 41] Surgical wound complication rates are 10% when a neck dissection is done 5 to 17 weeks after radio-chemotherapy, neck closure with pedicled flaps is required in 6% [42]. This could be another good reason to advocate neck dissection prior to radio-chemotherapy, which reduces wound complication rates to 2.5% [43]. The effect of radiation is also found to be dose dependent. Higher doses of radiation result in extensive fibrosis, hypoxia, and decreased leukocyte migration, which may be linked with higher infection rates [44]. In contrast, a study of 708 necks found no significant differences between previously irradiated cases and those undergoing surgery primarily [40]. During surgery, a subplatysmal plane should be the plane of choice to maximize skin flap blood supply. The incision of skin and raising of flaps should be done in stages, mainly if bilateral flaps are performed, as it further limits blood supply. It is also important to not allow skin flaps to desiccate. If the margins of the flap desiccate, then it may be necessary to excise 2–3 mm of edges. If a tracheotomy is to be concomitantly performed, neck dissection incision designs should be carefully planned. If tracheotomy is close to the incision, this can increase the risk of infection and impair drain suction upon closure. When closing the skin flaps, it is crucial to prevent dead space without increased tension on the wound and causing skin necrosis [42].

Management of Skin Incision Complications

Management of skin incision complications of neck dissections can be divided into conservative and invasive measures. The most common complications include dehiscence [deep and superficial], wound infection, flap necrosis, and aesthetic results, including hypertrophic scarring or keloids.

Wound dehiscence in a study of 708 neck dissections had 43 cases of epidermolysis, mostly in T-intersection areas of the incision, which were all treated successfully with a conservative approach. Eleven patients experienced deep dehiscence, five of which had to be managed with pedicle flaps. In the same study, there was a low rate of wound infections with only two patients, although all patients received 24-hour postoperative antibiotics. This low infection rate could be attributed to the extensive vascular supply to the neck and the uncontaminated nature of the neck as a surgical field; however, if there is contamination of the neck from the larynx, tracheostomy site, or salivary leak from the mouth, infections rates tend to increase. Previous radiotherapy had no adverse effect on wound infection [45]. A multitude of studies supports that radiation increases the risk of wound complications [40]. Closure technique can also be linked to dehiscence or infection rate. The use of staples was shown to be protective against surgical wound infections after the closure of total laryngectomies [41]. Utilizing staples for the closure of neck dissections showed efficacy by decreasing neck closure time, provided better aesthetics, minimal pain at removal, and faster healing when compared with sutures (Fig. 2.13). However, staples are approximately five times the expense of sutures, something that should be taken into consideration against prolonged operating time. Wound infections can also be prevented with enforcing aseptic techniques, such as proper

Fig. 2.13 Apron incision for a selective neck dissection closed with skin staples

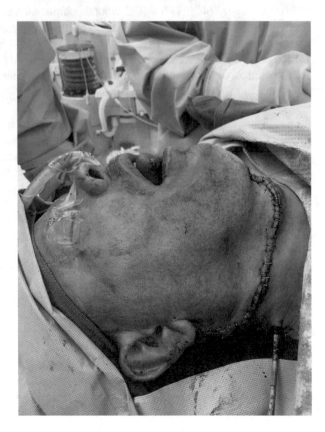

preparation of the surgical site to remove transient pathological bacteria and decrease resident flora counts. Removal of excess body hair may also reduce the risk of infection [41]. Limiting postoperative antibiotics lowers the risk of developing resistant bacteria [46]. Dehiscence in the setting of neck dissection can lead to disastrous results. The most feared complication is carotid blow out, which is associated with a 60% morbidity and 50% mortality. Emergency ligation surgery can result in hemiplegia, aphasia, and dysarthria.

Conservative Management

Conservative management of skin incision complications often results in wound healing by secondary intention. Several options can be used in conjunction to improve the chances of closure, including activity modification, diet modification, wound care, and pharmacologic methods, some of which have been mentioned previously. In most cases of dehiscence, flap necrosis and wound infections will heal with these interventions alone. However, deeper dehiscence or surgical wound infections may require more involved interventions, including surgical washouts or pedicled flaps for coverage.

Wet to Dry Therapy

Wet to dry therapy is considered a form of wound debridement that achieves essential goals to help with wound healing, as it eliminates necrotic tissues, exudates, bacteria, and their products while facilitating the natural healing process. The wet component of the debridement is achieved by placing a saline-damped gauze over the wound, where the dry part takes place when the gauze becomes dry and is subsequently removed. "Wet to dry" is a suitable option for moderate size defects where immediate repair is not possible because the neck being in the fleshy granulation phase of healing or due to patient-specific reasons. This technique has few drawbacks; first, it is labor-intensive when performed in the hospital setting and requires home care or family member education and participation. The second drawback is wet to dry debridement might be a painful process and might agitate the underlying bed of granulation tissue. In large neck wounds, wet to dry may serve as an initial or temporary measure until definitive treatment can be performed (Fig. 2.14).

Negative Pressure Wound Therapy [NPWT]

Negative pressure wound therapy has been shown to accelerate the wound healing process. Over the past 20 years, it has become an increasingly valuable tool for treating acute and chronic wounds, contaminated wounds, surgical dehiscence, fistulas, and other indications. Wound VAC therapy usually involves placing a porous sponge to wound bed, occlusive tape over the sponge, and tubing attached to a vacuum that provides negative pressure to the wound bed (Fig. 2.15). A canister is then attached to the vacuum then collects fluid from the bed. This treatment seems to be effective as it provides extraction of exudates from the wound

Fig. 2.14 Serial wet to
dry, until a granulation bed
was formed, and the skin
defect was covered with a
split-thickness skin graft

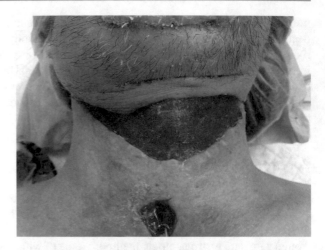

Fig. 2.15 NPWT applied
on the skin defect, for a
poorly controlled diabetic
patient

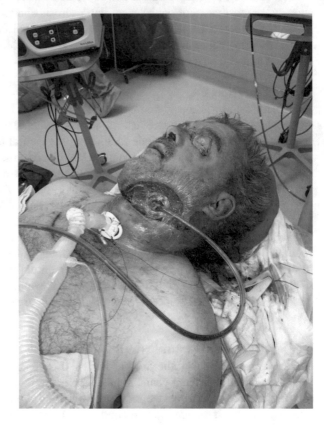

bed, decreases interstitial edema, increases vascularity to the wound bed, pro-
motes granulation tissue formation, decreases bacterial burden, stimulates fibro-
blasts/ endothelial cells, and assists with mechanical contracture of the wound

bed. There is strong evidence for the use of Wound VAC therapy in the post-surgical wound, although that specifically targeted towards the use of head and neck wounds is much more limited due to previous concern for application over complex topography, application on exposed great vessels, or use over previous free flap graft sites. Thus, indication for NPWT is not well defined in the head and neck. Although, in one institutional study of 115 patients with neck wounds status post head and neck surgery, they only experienced a 3.5% complication rate, demonstrating the safety of this strategy and establishing the use of this modality in the area of great vessels or free tissue transfer.

There is no specific regiment for use in head and neck wounds, although most of the reported regiments have verified the effectiveness of Wound VACs. Application is best managed under general anesthesia to provide sufficient comfort for the patient as well as an ideal placement of the vac for optimal results. In the author's experience, the Wound VAC settings are often placed at 125 mm Hg on continuous for optimal results. Wound VACs then require frequent changes around 2–3 times a week either in OR or bedside depending on wound characteristics, institutional policy, and patient performance. Wound VAC should be used until sufficient granulation has taken place to allow for either conventional wound care measures to take place or, ultimately, skin graft reconstruction [47]. Wound VAC Versflo technologies have been recently implemented into the head and neck wound care, and limited studies have been performed but show promising results. NPWTi is a modification of conventional NPWT as adjunctive therapy in the treatment of acute and chronic wounds. It provides the proven benefits of NPWT with controlled delivery of topical solutions such as irrigation cleansers, antiseptics, and antibiotics. This system introduces the extra substance through an additional tubing system when the VAC is not running. The foam and wound bed are then soaked in the desired fluid for a designated time, then taken back up through the Wound VAC. This process can be repeated as often as needed [48].

Closed Surgical Drains [CSD]

Suction drains are often placed in the setting of neck dissections at the time of surgery, especially if there is a concern for increased serosanguinous drainage, the development of hematoma, or chyle leak. Hemostasis should be achieved intra-operatively with either electrocautery or hemostatic agents. Despite meticulous intra-operatively, hemostasis drain placement might help preventing a hematoma formation. This can also help to decrease tension on incisions, diminish delayed wound healing, and reduce the risk of infection or flap necrosis [49]. While usage of suction drains is standard practice, some believe that drains should be removed promptly as they may lead to increased risk of infection, especially once the output is diminished, and minimal benefit is gained from leaving them. A systematic multidisciplinary review on the potential association of surgical site infections and closed suction drains demonstrated that judicious use and prompt, timely removal of CSDs should occur. Due to the scant evidence directly linking CSDs and surgical site infections, prophylactic antibiotics was not indicated with prolonged suction drains [50].

Invasive Measures

Sharp/Surgical Debridement

If conservative measures fail, surgical debridement is the next step; this encompasses sharp debridement using a variety of methods such as cold scalpel and scissors. This might be augmented with pulsed lavage, and care should be taken to avoid vascular structures or free flaps vascular pedicle. It is advised to debride any questionable skin; this will help to determine the final defect size.

Signs of adequate surgical debridement are cutting back to healthy bleeding tissues, when this is achieved, local flaps might be used if primary closure is not achievable. If both options fail, regional (Fig. 2.16) and free flaps might be used (Fig. 2.17).

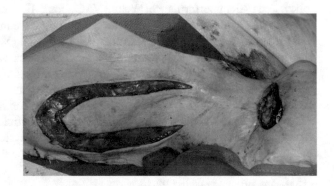

Fig. 2.16 Supraclavicular flap/regional flap used to cover a neck wound with plate exposure

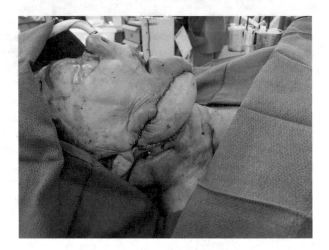

Fig. 2.17 A large neck defect covered with an anterolateral thigh flap

Surgical Management of Keloids/Hypertrophic Scars

In the setting of hypertrophic scarring, the timing of surgical treatment is vital for effective scar revision. These scars can mature for over a year, resulting in flattening and softening without any intervention. Therefore, surgical excision might not be required even though post-excision recurrence with hypertrophic scars is low. If scar contracture occurs, surgical intervention might assist in releasing contracture [51]; however, the same set of risk factors associated with skin complication after a neck dissection are shared with surgical management of hypertrophic scars /keloid formation and should be discussed thoroughly with the patient.

Management of hypertrophic scars starts with scar manipulation and massage to break the scar bands, silicone gel or sheeting, and scheduled injection with steroids every 6 weeks. Silicone sheeting offers an occlusive dressing that provides hydration to the stratum corneum and is an evidence-based adjunct to wound healing to prevent hypertrophic and keloid scars. It is generally utilized for a 6- to 12-month duration. Pulse dye laser can be used in conjunction with steroid injections to augments its effect. The mechanism of action is an inhibition of fibroblast production of collagen fibers, as well as inhibiting angiogenesis and often decreasing overall scar tissue formation [52].

References

1. Thiers BH, Maize JC, Spicer SS, Cantor AB. The effect of aging and chronic sun exposure on human Langerhans cell populations. J Invest Dermatol. 1984;82(3):223–6.
2. Gilchrest BA, Blog FB, Szabo G. Effects of aging and chronic sun exposure on melanocytes in human skin. J Invest Dermatol. 1979;73(2):141–3.
3. Shuster S, Black MM, McVitie E. The influence of age and sex on skin thickness, skin collagen and density. Br J Dermatol. John Wiley & Sons Ltd. 1975;93(6):639–43.
4. Gaboriau HP, Murakami CS. Skin anatomy and flap physiology. Otolaryngol Clin N Am. 2001;34(3):555–69.
5. Whetzel TP, Mathes SJ. Arterial anatomy of the face: an analysis of vascular territories and perforating cutaneous vessels. Plast Reconstr Surg. 1992;89(4):591–603–discussion604–5.
6. Granger HJ, Goodman AH, Granger DN. Role of resistance and exchange vessels in local microvascular control of skeletal muscle oxygenation in the dog. Circ Res. 1976;38(5):379–85.
7. Folkow B. Role of the nervous system in the control of vascular tone. Circulation. 1960;21(5):760–8.
8. Lucas JB. The physiology and biomechanics of skin flaps. Facial Plast Surg Clin North Am. 2017;25(3):303–11.
9. Taylor GI, Palmer JH. The vascular territories (angiosomes) of the body: experimental study and clinical applications. Br J Plast Surg. 1987;40(2):113–41.
10. Houseman ND, Taylor GI, Pan WR. The angiosomes of the head and neck: anatomic study and clinical applications. Plast Reconstr Surg. 2000;105(7):2287–313.
11. Rabson JA, Hurwitz DJ, Futrell JW. The cutaneous blood supply of the neck: relevance to incision planning and surgical reconstruction. Br J Plast Surg. 1985;38(2):208–19.
12. Grove GL. Age-related differences in healing of superficial skin wounds in humans. Arch Dermatol Res. 1982;272(3–4):381–5.

13. Montagna W, Carlisle K. Structural changes in ageing skin. Br J Dermatol 4 ed. 1990;122 Suppl 35(s35):61–70.
14. Divi V, Chen MM, Hara W, Shah D, Narvasa K, Segura Smith A, et al. Reducing the time from surgery to adjuvant radiation therapy: an institutional quality improvement project. Otolaryngol Head Neck Surg. 2018;159(1):158–65.
15. Chang P-H, Yeh K-Y, Huang J-S, Lai C-H, Wu T-H, Lan Y-J, et al. Pretreatment performance status and nutrition are associated with early mortality of locally advanced head and neck cancer patients undergoing concurrent chemoradiation. Eur Arch Otorhinolaryngol. 2012;270(6):1909–15.
16. Talwar B, Donnelly R, Skelly R, Donaldson M. Nutritional management in head and neck cancer: United Kingdom National Multidisciplinary Guidelines. J Laryngol Otol. 2016;130:S32–40.
17. Stadelmann WK, Digenis AG, Tobin GR. Physiology and healing dynamics of chronic cutaneous wounds. Am J Surg. 1998;176(2A Suppl):26S–38S.
18. Pellini R, Mercante G, Marchese C, Terenzi V, Sperduti I, Manciocco V, et al. Predictive factors for postoperative wound complications after neck dissection. Acta Otorhinolaryngol Ital. 2013;33(1):16–22.
19. Medina JE, Byers RM. Supraomohyoid neck dissection: rationale, indications, and surgical technique. Head Neck. John Wiley & Sons, Ltd. 1989;11(2):111–22.
20. Kerawala CJ, Heliotos M. Prevention of complications in neck dissection. Head Neck Oncol. BioMed Central. 2009;1(1):35–6.
21. Crile G. Landmark article Dec 1, 1906: excision of cancer of the head and neck. With special reference to the plan of dissection based on one hundred and thirty-two operations. By George Crile. JAMA. 1987;258:3286. 8 p.
22. Omura S, Bukawa H, Kawabe R, Aoki S, Fujita K. Comparison between hockey stick and reversed hockey stick incision: gently curved single linear neck incisions for oral cancer. Int J Oral Maxillofac Surg. 1999;28(3):197–202.
23. Macfee WF. Transverse incisions for neck dissection. Ann Surg. 1960;151(2):279–84.
24. Roy S, Shetty V, Sherigar V, Hegde P, Prasad R. Evaluation of four incisions used for radical neck dissection- a comparative study. Asian Pac J Cancer Prev. 2019;20(2):575–80.
25. Lahey FH, Hare HF, Warren S. Carcinoma of the thyroid. Ann Surg. 1940 Dec;112(6):977–1005.
26. Agrawal G, Gupta A, Choraria A, Tiwari S, Chaudhary V. Comparison of standard modified shrobingers incision versus transverse cervical incision for neck dissection – our experience. Otolaryngol Case Rep. Elsevier. 2018;6:47–50.
27. Shah JP. Patterns of cervical lymph node metastasis from squamous carcinomas of the upper aerodigestive tract. Am J Surg. 1990;160(4):405–9.
28. Kademani D, Dierks EJ. A straight-line incision for neck dissection: technical note. J Oral Maxillofac Surg. 2005;63(4):563–5.
29. Schobinger R. The use of a long anterior skin flap in radical neck resections. Ann Surg. 1957;146(2):221–3.
30. Attie JN. A single transverse incision for radical neck dissection. Surgery. 1957;41(3):498–502.
31. Gulati A, Shekar K, Downie IP. Aesthetic incision for neck dissection. Br J Oral Maxillofac Surg. 2012;50(2):183–4.
32. Yii NW, Patel SG, Williamson P, Breach NM. Use of apron flap incision for neck dissection. Plast Reconstr Surg. 1999;103(6):1655–60.
33. Chau JKM, Dzigielewski P, Mlynarek A, Cote DW, Allen H, Harris JR, et al. Steel scalpel versus electrocautery blade: comparison of cosmetic and patient satisfaction outcomes of different incision methods. J Otolaryngol Head Neck Surg. 2009;38(4):427–33.
34. Aird LNF, Brown CJ. Systematic review and meta-analysis of electrocautery versus scalpel for surgical skin incisions. Am J Surg. 2012;204(2):216–21.
35. Kuri M, Nakagawa M, Tanaka H, Hasuo S, Kishi Y. Determination of the duration of preoperative smoking cessation to improve wound healing after head and neck surgery. Anesthesiology. 2005;102(5):892–6.

36. Hatcher JL, Sterba KR, Tooze JA, Day TA, Carpenter MJ, Alberg AJ, et al. Tobacco use and surgical outcomes in patients with head and neck cancer. Head Neck. 2016;38(5):700–6.
37. Sørensen LT, Jørgensen T. Short-term pre-operative smoking cessation intervention does not affect postoperative complications in colorectal surgery: a randomized clinical trial. Color Dis. 2003;5(4):347–52.
38. Yang GP, Longaker MT. Abstinence from smoking reduces incisional wound infection: a randomized, controlled trial. Ann Surg. 2003;238(1):6–8.
39. Kerawala C, Brennan PA, Cascarini L, Godden D, Coombes D, McCaul J. Management of tumour spillage during parotid surgery for pleomorphic adenoma. Br J Oral Maxillofac Surg British Association of Oral and Maxillofacial Surgeons. 2014;52(1):3–6.
40. Genden EM, Ferlito A, Shaha AR, Talmi YP, Robbins KT, Rhys-Evans PH, et al. Complications of neck dissection. Acta Otolaryngol. 2003;123(7):795–801.
41. Aires FT, Dedivitis RA, Castro MAF, Bernardo WM, Cernea CR, Brandão LG. Efficacy of stapler pharyngeal closure after total laryngectomy: a systematic review. Head Neck. 2014;36(5):739–42.
42. Ha PK, Couch ME, Tufano RP, Koch WM, Califano JA. Short hospital stay after neck dissection. Otolaryngol Head Neck Surg. 2005;133(5):677–80.
43. Prades JM, Timoshenko AP, Schmitt TH, Delolme MP, Francoz M, Martin C, et al. Planned neck dissection before combined chemoradiation for pyriform sinus carcinoma. Acta Otolaryngol. 2008;128(3):324–8.
44. Mathes SJ, Alexander J. Radiation injury. Surg Oncol Clin NA. 1996;5(4):809–24.
45. Coskun H, Erisen L, Basut O. Factors affecting wound infection rates in head and neck surgery. Otolaryngol Head Neck Surg. 2000;123(3):328–33.
46. Flynn TR, Halpern LR. Antibiotic selection in head and neck infections. Oral Maxillofac Surg Clin NA. 2003;15(1):17–38.
47. O'Malley QF, Sims JR, Sandler ML, Spitzer H, Urken ML. The use of negative pressure wound therapy in the primary setting for high-risk head and neck surgery. Am J Otolaryngol. 2020;41:102470.
48. Back DA, Scheuermann-Poley C, Willy C. Recommendations on negative pressure wound therapy with instillation and antimicrobial solutions - when, where and how to use: what does the evidence show? Int Wound J. 2013;10 Suppl 1(s1):32–42.
49. Kreutzer K, Storck K, Weitz J. Current evidence regarding prophylactic antibiotics in head and neck and maxillofacial surgery. Biomed Res Int. 2014;2014(12):879437.
50. Reiffel AJ, Barie PS, Spector JA. A multi-disciplinary review of the potential association between closed-suction drains and surgical site infection. Surg Infect. 2013;14(3):244–69.
51. Gauglitz GG. Management of keloids and hypertrophic scars: current and emerging options. Clin Cosmet Investig Dermatol. 2013;6:103–14.
52. Khan MA, Bashir MM, Khan FA. Intralesional triamcinolone alone and in combination with 5-fluorouracil for the treatment of keloid and hypertrophic scars. J Pak Med Assoc. 2014;64(9):1003–7.

Infectious Complications

Lindsay L. Graves and Thomas Schlieve

Definitions, Epidemiology, and Risk Factors

Surgical site infection (SSI), as defined by the Centers for Disease Control (CDC)'s National Healthcare Safety Network (NHSN) and American College of Surgeons ACS National Surgical Quality Improvement Program (ACS-NSQIP), is an infectious process occurring at the incisions, organs, or space at the location of previous surgery within 30 days post-procedure. The presence of only one of the following is required for the designation of a process to be an infection: purulent drainage, abscess on clinical exam or by imaging, organisms identified from an aseptically obtained specimen from the site, or an opened wound with localized tenderness, swelling, erythema, or heat. SSIs are further divided into the categories of superficial incisional infection, deep incisional infection, and organ/space infection. Stitch abscess is not considered to be an SSI. In the case of neck surgeries, the following specific events are recognized: superficial incisional primary, deep incisional primary, ear/mastoid infection, oral cavity infection, and upper respiratory infection/pharyngitis/laryngitis/epiglottitis. Superficial infections are those that involve only the skin and subcutaneous soft tissues at the incision, while deep infections involve the deeper soft tissues (i.e., fascia, muscle), and organ/space infections may involve any part of the body deeper than the fascia and muscle layers [1, 2].

L. L. Graves (✉)
Department of Oral and Maxillofacial Surgery, Parkland Memorial Hospital,
Dallas, TX, USA
e-mail: Lindsay.Graves@phhs.org

T. Schlieve
Department of Surgery, Division of Oral and Maxillofacial Surgery, UT Southwestern
Medical Center, Parkland Memorial Hospital, Texas Health – Dallas Presbyterian,
Dallas, TX, USA
e-mail: Thomas.Schlieve@utsouthwestern.edu

© Springer Nature Switzerland AG 2021
T. Schlieve, W. Zaid (eds.), *Complications in Neck Dissection*,
https://doi.org/10.1007/978-3-030-62739-3_3

Incidence values of SSI after neck dissection (ND-SSI) differ between the NSQIP data and various studies. In an analysis of the NSQIP database numbers from 2006 to 2011 (n = 9462 patients), Jain et al. found of rate of 2–9%, while pre-existing literature ranged from 3% to 38% [3]. In a prospective study of 79 patients, the rate was found to be 15% [4]. A retrospective cohort study of 370 patients found an incidence of 19.7%, and further stratified the infections by type; 54.8% of infections were deep incisional, 24.7% superficial, and 20.5% organ/space in the neck dissection postoperative bed [5].

Patient, site, and operative factors can be predictive of an increased propensity for ND-SSI. American Society of Anesthesiologists (ASA) status ≥3, cardiovascular disease and neurologic disease have been shown to be risk factors. Male sex was shown to be an independent risk factor in one study [5], however, was not in another. Interestingly, preoperative diagnosis of diabetes does not appear to be associated with increased SSI rate [6]. Perhaps a known diagnosis of diabetes allows for preoperative optimization. Not particular to neck dissection, but in head and neck oncologic procedures in general, low preoperative serum albumin, a marker of malnutrition, is a predictor of SSI and a poor prognostic indicator overall [7]. Cancer stage had no association. Previous radiotherapy was not associated with increased risk of infection; however, it was associated with more severe infections [6].

Longer operative times (>7 h), increased blood loss, oropharyngeal contamination, and presence of tracheostomy put the patient at higher risk [3–5]. Thoracic duct severance and subsequent chyle leak, which occurs in 1–2.5% of neck dissections, especially when operating on the left side, has also been identified a risk factor. This is theoretically due to spillage of lymphocytes and immunoglobulins resulting in decreased immune function [8]. Certain procedures, such as radical and extended dissections, bilateral dissection, and concurrent reconstruction with pedicled flap, increase risk, but also certainly increase operative time [4, 9]. It is not known if the addition of neck dissection to the ablative surgery increases risk for SSI; however, a study out of MD Anderson did show that N stage was predictive, calling into question if this was due to the metastatic disease itself or the treatment [10]. A more recent study, specifically of laryngectomies, found that the addition of neck dissection did not result in increased complication rate [11]. However, it is indisputable that adding neck dissection to the procedure list significantly prolongs the total surgical time, thereby increasing risk of SSI indirectly.

Pathogens

A variety of organisms are responsible for ND-SSI. In a 2016 retrospective cohort study, of 73 patients who developed SSI, 60 showed positive cultures; 48.3% grew a polymicrobial flora. Gram-positive organisms were present in 51.5% of cultures, and Gram-negatives in 43.5%. Unsurprisingly, the common skin organism *Staphylococcus aureus* played a part in 32.6% of the infections, with 93.3% of these being methicillin-resistant (MRSA). Candida was present in 5.4% of cultures. *Klebsiella pneumoniae*, ubiquitous in the mouth, skin, and intestines, and also a common nosocomial pathogen, was the second most common individual bacterium present in 14.1% of cases. Of these, 30.8% and 53.8% were cefotaxime and ciprofloxacin resistant, respectively. *Pseudomonas aeruginosa*, well known to be an opportunist of the airway and wounds, was found in 12.0%. *Enterococcus* genus, generally commensals of the digestive tract, comprised 2% of infections [5]. Given this broad range of players, empiric coverage for prophylaxis and treatment of ND-SSI should be equally broad and when possible, directed by cultures.

Antibiotic Prophylaxis

The CDC has published guidelines regarding antibiotic prophylaxis for all surgeries in general. Strong and well-evidenced "Category I" recommendations will be reviewed:

- Patients should shower or bathe with soap or antiseptic on at least the night before planned operation.
- Parenteral antibiotics should be given time such that bactericidal concentrations will be obtained locally prior to the incision start. Generally, this is within 1 h, vancomycin can be given up to 2 h in advance, as it should be given slowly to avoid hypotension [12]. In clean and clean-contaminated procedures, prophylactic parenteral antibiotics need not be re-dosed after closure within the operating room.
- Other than the use of intraoperative skin, preparation with an alcohol-based antiseptic prior to incision start, nonparenteral (e.g., ointments, solutions, powders) antibiotics should not be applied to the incision site.
- Perioperative glycemic control with target blood glucose less than 200 mg/dL in both diabetic and nondiabetic patients is recommended. There is insufficient evidence to recommend a specific target hemoglobin A1c (used to estimate the average blood glucose of a patient over time).
- Increased FiO2 air (unless contraindicated) should be given during surgery and after extubation for a period of time. Adequate volume replacement and normothermia promote tissue oxygen delivery [13].

Specific to the head and neck, for clean procedures such as isolated neck dissection, antimicrobial prophylaxis is not necessary because the frequency of SSI is less than 1% without prophylaxis [14], and no benefits are seen [9]. However, prophylaxis should be considered in the case of anticipated lengthy operative time [15].

In the case of drain placement or other prosthetic material, cefazolin or cefuroxime (or clindamycin if patient is allergic to beta-lactams) can be given prophylactically. In this case, the presumed colonizers are the skin flora: *Staphylococcus aureus, S. epidermidis,* and *streptococci*. Cefazolin is generally preferred over cefuroxime due to increasing resistance of *S. aureus*. In areas of high prevalence of methicillin-resistant *Staphylococcus aureus* (MRSA), or in a patient who is a known carrier, vancomycin is the best choice [12]. Clindamycin may also be used in this case, though the local anti-bio-gram should be consulted due to increasing prevalence of resistance. In a single-site study from Vanderbilt in Nashville, Tennessee, the proportion of clindamycin-resistant *Staph* rose steadily from 12.2% to 40.0% within a 4-year period [16]. Clindamycin is also associated with a higher odds ratio of short-term complications (SSI, dehiscence, and antibiotic-associated complications) when compared to other regimens [17]. No matter the regimen chooses, an antibiotic duration of 24 h postoperatively is generally sufficient; extending coverage until drain removal has not shown benefit [15]. A full list of regimens for clean head and neck procedures with prosthetic material placement is listed in Table 3.1.

Most neck dissections are clean-contaminated due to either violation of the oral or pharyngeal mucosa by the tumor itself, need for adequate surgical margins during resection, or presence of a tracheostomy tube. The incidence of SSI without prophylaxis in this group is much higher (24–78%) [19]. Current practice guidelines, put forth by the Infectious Diseases Society of America (IDSA), the Surgical Infection Society (SIS), the American Society of Health Systems Pharmacists (ASHSP), and the Society for Healthcare Epidemiology of America (SHEA) for clean-contaminated procedures of the head and neck, call for antibiotics to be given within 1 h before incision and stopped 24 h after wound closure. Antibiotics of choice include cefazolin or cefuroxime plus metronidazole, ampicillin/sulbactam, or clindamycin for the beta-lactam allergic (see Table 3.2) [20]. This coverage considers skin flora plus anerobes and enteric gram-negative bacilli. The duration of 24 h, opposed to a prolonged course, has been validated in multiple recent systematic reviews and metaanalyses [20, 21]. Theoretically, short-course regimens also decrease the likelihood of development of antibiotic-resistant strains, decrease potential for medication-related adverse events, and lower hospital costs [21].

The use of topical forms of antibiotic prophylaxis has been studied in patients who have undergone major head and neck oncologic surgery, but this is not standard practice. One group out of Japan found reduction in SSI incidence when tetracycline ointment was applied to the dorsum of the tongue every 6 h for the first 48 h postoperatively [22]. Another study showed benefit using clindamycin mouthwash preoperatively, irrigation intraoperatively, and mouthwash again postoperatively for patients undergoing laryngectomy with neck dissection [23]. However, yet another

Table 3.1 Common antibiotic prophylactic regimens for clean head and neck procedures with prosthetic material placement (i.e., a drain)[a] [12, 18]

Antibiotic	Dosing and route	Re-dose interval
Cefazolin	<120 kg: 2 g IV, ≥120 kg: 3 g IV	4 h
Cefuroxime	1.5 g IV	4 h
Vancomycin	15 mg/kg (max 2 g)	N/A
Clindamycin	900 mg IV 300 mg PO	N/A
Cephalexin	500 mg PO	N/A

[a]Note that these values assume normal renal function for drug clearance. Dose and re-dose timing adjustment may need to be altered in the setting of reduced glomerular filtration rate (GFR)

Table 3.2 Common antibiotic prophylactic regimens for clean-contaminated head and neck procedures[a] [12, 18]

Antibiotic	Dosing and route	Re-dose interval
Cefazolin -or-	<120 kg: 2 g IV, ≥120 kg: 3 g IV	4 h
Cefuroxime -or-	1.5 g IV	4 h
Vancomycin -PLUS-	15 mg/kg (max 2 g)	N/A
Metronidazole -or-	500 mg IV	N/A
Gentamicin -or-	5 mg/kg IV	
Aztreonam -or-	2 g IV	
Levofloxacin -or-	500 mg IV	
Ciprofloxacin	400 mg IV	
Ampicillin-sulbactam	3 g IV	2 h
Clindamycin	900 mg IV	6 h

[a]Note that these values assume normal renal function for drug clearance. Dose and re-dose timing adjustment may need to be altered in the setting of reduced glomerular filtration rate (GFR)

study of piperacillin-tazobactam prior to surgery and daily for 2 days postoperatively did not demonstrate added benefit when added to the standard parenteral prophylactic regimen [24].

Other Forms of Mitigation

Surgical technique can also be used to reduce infection rate. Contamination can be minimized by separation of the oropharyngeal and neck dissection fields, if possible, given previously the described tumor and operative factors. Treatment can be staged when feasible, separating excisional and neck dissection phases by time. Additionally, judicious use of soft issue flaps may aid in the mitigation of SSIs through minimization of dead space, provision of anatomic barriers, and improvement in surgical bed vascularity [3].

Drain placement, either a closed suction type (i.e., Jackson-Pratt) or passive (i.e., red rubber catheter), is often utilized by head and neck surgeons following neck dissection to prevent postoperative hematoma, seroma, and dead space. These occurrences may provide nidus for infection or compromise vascularity of skin flaps, leading to necrosis and subsequent infection; 86% of surveyed surgeons routinely place a drain after selective neck dissection. However, drain placement may in and of itself be a contributing factor to infection, as it is a foreign body and, by design, breeches the skin, creating a pathway from the skin surface to the wound interior. Suction drains may damage tissues causing areas of necrosis that serve to harbor and feed bacteria [25]. It has been shown that prolonged drainage, especially if the patient is discharged home with the drain, leads to increased risk of surgical site infection [26–28].

Because of this, it is prudent to remove a drain as soon as it is no longer needed; for, at this time, the risk-to-benefit ratio may be reversed. The most commonly used criterion for removal is less than 25–30 mL output within 24 h. This value is somewhat arbitrary, and studies have questioned if this guideline should be modified in order to reduce the length of time of drain use [29]. Additionally, earlier drain discontinuation will often shorten hospital length of stay, which decreases risk of exposure to nosocomial pathogens. One study found that a threshold of less than 100 mL in 24 h resulted in decreased mean hospital length of stay without concomitant increase in complication rate, when compared to the traditional cutoff of less than 30 mL in 24 h [30]. Other studies have questioned not only the volume but also the time component of this measure. The highest rate of drainage has been shown to occur during the first 8 h postoperatively. Knowing that drainage rate decreases with time, a new criterion of a drainage rate of ≤ 1 mL/h over 8-h intervals was shown to result in more discharges within 24 h and no increase in complications [31–33]. The utilization of prophylactic postoperative antibiotics until drain removal, as previously stated, has not been shown to be efficacious [15].

Recognition

As previously discussed, surgical site infections after neck dissection present with the famed cardinal signs of inflammation: *rubor, calor, dolor, tumor*. Purulence may or may not be evident clinically or on imaging based on stage of infection and depth (superficial, deep, or organ/space.) Compared to other SSIs elsewhere, those in the head and neck appear to be more often deep incisional or organ/space, so it may be prudent to obtain imaging early if there is any suspicion of infection. The same retrospective cohort study found that median time from surgery to diagnosis of SSI was 12 days, with a range of 1–19 days, and 71.2% occurring within the first 14 days [5]. Some advocate for SSI surveillance using wound fluid drainage sampling, based on the findings that negative culture of drainage at postoperative day 3 had a negative predictive value of 96% for subsequent SSI4, and elevated TNF-alpha, IL-1, IL-6 levels can herald SSI before clinical signs and symptoms [34]. While these are interesting findings, they have yet to be studied extensively and put into routine clinical practice.

Management

Should SSI after neck dissection occur, treatment consists of empiric antibiotics, wound and blood cultures, and surgical debridement and wash out. Based on the most common pathogens isolated from necks with SSI, vancomycin and antipseudomonal penicillin or cephalosporin should be started as initial therapy and narrowed after culture speciation and sensitivities are available [5].

Necrotizing SSI

Cases of necrotizing fasciitis at the site of previous neck dissection have been described [35, 36]. This rapidly progressing infection of the subcutaneous tissues and superficial fascia is generally seen in the extremities or genital region, and rarely affects the head and neck [37]. Even then, it is usually due to odontogenic, tonsillar, or pharyngeal primary infection, not SSI [38]. It generally presents as a sudden increase in local pain, with increasing erythema of the skin that progresses to dusky cyanosis and subsequent skin breakdown. Crepitus can be present if the causative organisms are gas producing. Diagnosis is clinical, based on appearance and timeline. If suspected, the patient should immediately be placed on high-dose, broad-spectrum antibiotics, and urgently taken to the operating room for extensive local debridement and irrigation to avoid certain progression to sepsis and death. Multiple sessions of debridement are usually needed [37]. Maggot therapy has been used successfully as an alternative, especially in the critically ill patient who may not survive repeat anesthesia and surgery, with the potential advantage of antibiotic enzymes in their saliva and improved wound healing [35].

Outcomes

Given proper management, most patients will have improvement within a week (82.2%). Death despite treatment results in approximately 1% of cases [5]. Oddly enough, however, in one retrospective study of 201 head and neck cancer patients, the 5-year survival rate of the group who had SSI was higher than the control group (44% vs. 31%). SSI appeared to be most beneficial in stage 3 disease. It is theorized that bacterial contamination triggers immune system activation, acting as an adjuvant immunotherapy; however, this has yet to be substantiated and remains controversial [39].

Carotid Blowout

Carotid blowout syndrome (CBS) is an uncommon and dreaded sequela of head and neck cancer and its treatment. It occurs when the arterial wall is weakened and cannot withstand the outward force of the patient's blood pressure within. Overall incidence in patients who received major oncologic head and neck surgery is 3–4.5%. Previous irradiation to the area increases the risk dramatically due to diminished blood supply to the arterial wall, adventitial fibrosis, and premature atherosclerosis. Neck dissection predisposes a patient to CBS because of the removal of surrounding supportive tissues and stripping of the carotid sheath [40]. SSI after neck dissection further compounds the risk because of tissue necrosis and/or pharyngocutaneous fistula formation. Resultant local inflammatory products cause thrombosis of the vasa vasorum, compromising wall blood supply. Necrosis of the skin also diminishes perfusion and exposes the carotid to air if the overlying flap is lost, thereby causing desiccation. Exposure to salivary enzymes through a pharyngocutaneous fistula results in digestion of the arterial wall [40, 41]. Additionally, it should be noted that internal jugular vein rupture has been reported secondarily to thrombosis after infection of the dissected neck [42].

Half of patients with CBS will have a sentinel bleed, while the other half give no warning prior to massive hemorrhage. Treatment of this acutely life-threatening condition consists of emergent endovascular therapy or surgical ligation. Even with treatment, only about 50% of patients survive. Of those that do survive, 70% have resultant long-term neurologic morbidity [40].

Financial Burden

The occurrence of NS-SSI has profound impact on the patient as well our healthcare system. On average, length of stay (LOS) increases by 10 days from mean LOS for patients who underwent radical neck dissection. The mean charge per hospitalization for neck dissection without significant complication was $75,654 in 2008. An average increase of $77,826 per patient admission with SSI was found, and this further increased to $98,854 if penicillin-resistant organisms were involved [43].

Conclusion

In conclusion, surgical site infection after neck dissection is an uncommon occurrence. This is largely due to its preventative nature with standardized infection control practice and use of empiric prophylactic antibiotics in the perioperative period. If it occurs, it is generally very treatable with aggressive antibiotic therapy and surgical intervention. However, it has the potential for significant patient and healthcare system morbidity.

References

1. CDC, NHSN: CDC/NHSN Surveillance Definitions for Specific Types of Infections. Surveillance Definitions, 2020 https://www.cdc.gov.
2. Khuri SF, Henderson WG, Daley J, Jonasson O, Jones RS, et al. Successful implementation of the Department of Veterans Affairs' National Surgical Quality Improvement Program in the private sector: the Patient Safety in Surgery study. Ann Surg. 2008;248:329–36.
3. Jain U, Somerville J, Saha S, Hackett NJ, Ver Halen JP, Antony AK, Samant S. Oropharyngeal contamination predisposes to complications after neck dissection: an analysis of 9462 patients. Otolaryngol Head Neck Surg. 2015;153:71.
4. Candau-Alvarez A, Linares-Sicilia MJ, Dean-Ferrer A, Pérez-Navero JL. Role of culture of postoperative drainage fluid in the prediction of infection of the surgical site after major oncological operations of the head and neck. Br J Oral Maxillofac Surg. 2015;53:200.
5. Park SY, Kim MS, Eom JS, Lee JS, Rho YS. Risk factors and etiology of surgical site infection after radical neck dissection in patients with head and neck cancer. Korean J Intern Med. 2016;31:162.

6. Righi M, Manfredi R, Farneti G, Pasquini E, Cenacchi V. Short-term versus long-term antimicrobial prophylaxis in oncologic head and neck surgery. Head Neck. 1996;18:399.
7. Viasus D, Garcia-Vidal C, Simonetti A, Manresa F, Dorca J, Gudiol F, Carratalà J. Prognostic value of serum albumin levels in hospitalized adults with community-acquired pneumonia. J Infect. 2013;66:415.
8. Chen CY, Chen YH, Shiau EL, Liang HL, Chang HS, Chen HC. Therapeutic role of ultrasound-guided intranodal lymphangiography in refractory cervical chylous leakage after neck dissection: report of a case and review of the literature. Head Neck. 2016;38:E54.
9. Man LX, Beswick DM, Johnson JT. Antibiotic prophylaxis in uncontaminated neck dissection. Laryngoscope. 2011;121:1473.
10. Robbins KT, Favrot S, Hanna D, Cole R. Risk of wound infection in patients with head and neck cancer. Head Neck. 1990;12:143.
11. Xiao Y, Yuan S, Liu F, Liu B, Zhu J, He W, Li W, Kan Q. Comparison between wait-and-see policy and elective neck dissection in clinically N0 cutaneous squamous cell carcinoma of head and neck. Medicine. 2018;97:e10782.
12. Bratzler DW, Dellinger EP, Olsen KM, Perl TM, Auwaerter PG, Bolon MK, Fish DN, Napolitano LM, Sawyer RG, Slain D, Steinberg JP, Weinstein RA. Clinical practice guidelines for antimicrobial prophylaxis in surgery. Am J Health Syst Pharm. 2013;70:195.
13. Berriós-Torres SI, Umscheid CA, Bratzler DW, Leas B, Stone EC, Kelz RR, Reinke CE, Morgan S, Solomkin JS, Mazuski JE, Dellinger EP, Itani KMF, Berbari EF, Segreti J, Parvizi J, Blanchard J, Allen G, Kluytmans JAJW, Donlan R, Schecter WP. Centers for disease control and prevention guideline for the prevention of surgical site infection. JAMA Surg. 2017;152:784.
14. Slattery WH, Stringer SP, Cassisi NJ. Prophylactic antibiotic use in clean, uncontaminated neck dissection. Laryngoscope. 1995;105:244.
15. Fairbanks DNF. Pocket guide to antimicrobial therapy in otolaryngology-head and neck surgery. 3rd ed. Alexandria: AAOHNS; 2007.
16. Border M, Coke D, Lin SI. Increased incidence of clindamycin-resistance in head and neck infections within Oral and maxillofacial surgery. J Oral Maxillofac Surg. 2017;75:e379.
17. Langerman A, Ham SA, Pisano J, Pariser J, Hohmann SF, Meltzer DO. Laryngectomy complications are associated with perioperative antibiotic choice. Otolaryngol Head Neck Surg. 2015;153:60.
18. Antimicrobial prophylaxis for surgery. Med Lett Drugs Ther. 2016;58(1495):63–8.
19. Simo R, French G. The use of prophylactic antibiotics in head and neck oncological surgery. Curr Opin Otolaryngol Head Neck Surg. 2006;14:55.
20. Vila PM, Zenga J, Jackson RS. Antibiotic prophylaxis in clean-contaminated head and neck surgery: a systematic review and meta-analysis. Otolaryngol Head Neck Surg. 2017;157:580.
21. Oppelaar MC, Zijtveld C, Kuipers S, Ten Oever J, Honings J, Weijs W, Wertheim HFL. Evaluation of prolonged vs short courses of antibiotic prophylaxis following ear, nose, throat, and oral and maxillofacial surgery: a systematic review and meta-analysis. JAMA Otolaryngol Head Neck Surg. 2019;145:610.
22. Funahara M, Funahara S, Yanamoton M, Umeda M, Ueda T, Suzuki Y, Ota Y, Nishimaki F, Kurita H, Yamakawa N, Kirita T, Okura M, Mekaru Y, Arakaki K. Prevention of surgical site infection after oral cancer surgery by topical tetracycline. Medicine. 2017;96:e8891.
23. Grandis JR, Vickers RM, Rihs JD, Yu VL, Wagner RL, Kachman KK, Johnson JT. The efficacy of topical antibiotic prophylaxis for contaminated head and neck surgery. Laryngoscope. 1994;104:719.
24. Simons JP, Johnson JT, Yu VL, Vickers RM, Gooding WE, Myers EN, Pou AM, Wagner RL, Grandis JR. The role of topical antibiotic prophylaxis in patients undergoing contaminated head and neck surgery with flap reconstruction. Laryngoscope. 2001;111:329.
25. Amir I, Morar P, Belloso A. Postoperative drainage in head and neck surgery. Ann R Coll Surg Engl. 2010;92:651.

26. Barbadoro P, Marmorale C, Recanatini C, Mazzarini G, Pellegrini I, D'Errico MM, Prospero E. May the drain be a way in for microbes in surgical infections? Am J Infect Control. 2016;44:283.
27. Tian J, Li L, Liu P, Wang X. Comparison of drain versus no-drain thyroidectomy: a meta-analysis. Eur Arch Otorhinolaryngol. 2017;274:567.
28. Felippe WAB, Werneck GL, Santoro-Lopes G. Surgical site infection among women discharged with a drain in situ after breast cancer surgery. World J Surg. 2007;31:2293.
29. Hemmat SM, Wang SJ, Ryan WR. Neck dissection technique commonality and variance: a survey on neck dissection technique preferences among head and neck oncologic surgeons in the American Head and Neck Society. Int Arch Otorhinolaryngol. 2017, 21:8.
30. Tamplen ML, Tamplen J, Shuman E, Heaton CM, George JR, Wang SJ, Ryan WR. Comparison of output volume thresholds for drain removal after selective lateral neck dissection: a randomized clinical trial. JAMA Otolaryngol Head Neck Surg. 2017;143:1195.
31. Weiss E, McClelland P, Krupp J, Karadsheh M, Brady MS. Use of prolonged prophylactic antibiotics with closed suction drains in ventral abdominal hernia repair. Am Surg. 2019;85:403.
32. Urquhart JC, Collings D, Nutt L, Kuska L, Gurr KR, Siddiqi F, Rasoulinejad P, Fleming A, Collie J, Bailey CS. The effect of prolonged postoperative antibiotic administration on the rate of infection in patients undergoing posterior spinal surgery requiring a closed-suction drain: a randomized controlled trial. J Bone Joint Surg Am. 2019;101:1732.
33. Phillips BT, Fourman MS, Bishawi M, Zegers M, O'Hea BJ, Ganz JC, Huston TL, Dagum AB, Khan SU, Bui DT. Are prophylactic postoperative antibiotics necessary for immediate breast reconstruction? Results of a prospective randomized clinical trial. J Am Coll Surg. 2016;222:1116.
34. Candau-Alvarez A, Gil-Campos M, La Torre-Aguilar MJ De, Llorente-Cantarero F, Lopez-Miranda J, Perez-Navero JL. Early modification in drainage of interleukin-1β and tumor necrosis factor-α best predicts surgical-site infection after cervical neck dissection for oral cancer. J Oral Maxillofac Surg. 2015;73:1189.
35. Preuss SF, Stenzel MJ, Esriti A. The successful use of maggots in necrotizing fasciitis of the neck: a case report. Head Neck. 2004;26:747.
36. Danic Hadzibegovic A, Sauerborn D, Grabovac S, Matic I, Danic D. Necrotizing fasciitis of the neck after total laryngectomy. Eur Arch Otorhinolaryngol. 2013;270:277.
37. Misiakos EP, Bagias G, Patapis P, Sotiropoulos D, Kanavidis P, Machairas A. Current concepts in the management of necrotizing fasciitis. Front Surg. 2014;1:36.
38. Bloching M, Gudziol S, Gajda M, Berghaus A. Diagnose und Behandlung der nekrotisierenden Fasziitis in der Kopf-Hals-Region. TT – [Diagnosis and treatment of necrotizing fasciitis of the head and neck region]. Laryngorhinootologie. 2000;79:774.
39. Schantz SP, Skolnik EM, O'Neill JV. Improved survival associated with postoperative wound infection in laryngeal cancer: an analysis of its therapeutic implications. Otolaryngol Head Neck Surg. 1980;88:412.
40. Suárez C, Fernández-Alvarez V, Hamoir M, Mendenhall WM, Strojan P, Quer M, Silver CE, Rodrigo JP, Rinaldo A, Ferlito A. Carotid blowout syndrome: modern trends in management. Cancer Manag Res. 2018;10:5617.
41. Powitzky R, Vasan N, Krempl G, Medina J. Carotid blowout in patients with head and neck cancer. Ann Otol Rhinol Laryngol. 2010;119:476.
42. Ota Y, Aoki T, Karakida K, Miyasaka M. A case of rupture of the internal jugular vein caused by postoperative infection of functional neck dissection. Tokai J Exp Clin Med. 2001;26:123–5.
43. Lee MK, Dodson TB, Karimbux NY, Nalliah RP, Allareddy V. Effect of occurrence of infection-related never events on length of stay and hospital charges in patients undergoing radical neck dissection for head and neck cancer. Oral Surg Oral Med Oral Pathol Oral Radiol. 2013;116:147.

Complications Related to Lymphatics and Chyle Leak

4

Waleed Zaid, Peter Park, Beomjune Kim, and Rob Laughlin

Introduction

In this chapter, we discuss complications related to lymphatics and chyle leaks that occur during neck dissection procedures happening mainly at the left neck. It is beneficial to understand the anatomy of the lymphatic system, starting with embryology of the lymphatic system while emphasizing on the thoracic duct variations in its origin, course, and termination. Next, we discuss common drainage patterns of various anatomic subsites of the head and neck, and finally, we discuss the complications that might arise from developing a chyle leak, management of chyle, including medical and surgical management.

Embryology

Embryology of the lymphatic system shares some standard features with the venous system. Generally speaking, the development of the lymphatic system starts at six weeks of development from hemangioblastic stem cells, lymphatic clefts and sacs form around large veins [1] with blunt buds, at the end of the embryonic period there are six lymphatics sacs which are essentially pouch-like outgrowths of the endothelial layer, these sacs inherit their name from their corresponding anatomic locations, two jugular sacs, two iliac sacs, a single retroperitoneal lymph sac, and one cisterna chyli. Interconnected lymphatic capillaries with tissue channels act like a lymph collecting system from the initial lymphatic capillary concluding into the venous system. The histology of lymphatic

W. Zaid (✉) · P. Park · B. Kim · R. Laughlin
Oral and Maxillofacial Surgery Department, Louisiana State University Health Sciences Center, New Orleans, LA, USA
e-mail: wzaid@lsuhsc.edu; epark1@lsuhsc.edu; beomjune.kim@ctca-hope.com; rlaugh@lsuhsc.edu

© Springer Nature Switzerland AG 2021
T. Schlieve, W. Zaid (eds.), *Complications in Neck Dissection*,
https://doi.org/10.1007/978-3-030-62739-3_4

capillaries consists of a single layer of flat endothelial cells, with a thin basement membrane contributing to the greater permeability of the lymphatic system, particularly large molecules such as protein-rich fluid frequently located in the intercellular space. An additional histological feature of lymphatic capillaries is that they have numerous one-way valves, which preclude backflow. Occasionally the valves are very close to each other, contributing to the beaded appearance that lymphatic vessels might have. These lymphatic sacs degrade into groups of lymph nodes at 9 weeks of life, with simultaneous regression of many other lymphoid tissues. When the collected fluid, which made of electrolytes, fat-soluble vitamins, trace elements, and the glucose absorbed from the interstitial fluid, enters the lymphatic vessels, it is called lymph. It also transports proteins that cannot get past intestinal capillaries fenestration, chyle, or chylomicrons composed of monoglycerides and fatty acids, with cholesterol formed as a result of the breakdown of long-chain fatty acids by the bile salts [2]. An additional crucial function of lymph is carrying immune cells from the lymph nodes back to the systemic vascular circulation. Finally, the lymphatic system collects antigens from microorganisms close to their port of entry where these lymph nodes are heavily located to load an adaptive immune response. The lymphatic fluid movement in the lymphatic vessels occurs due to the contraction of the perilymphatic smooth muscles as well as applied pressure from adjacent musculoskeletal tissues [3]. The lymphatic vessels can be classified into afferent lymphatic vessels that drain into the lymph nodes and efferent lymphatic vessels that drain out of the lymph nodes. At the same time, this classification might look simple on its surface; sometimes, efferent lymphatic vessels from a lymph node might act as afferent to another lymph node.

Anatomy of the Thoracic Duct

The cisterna chyli, which is the abdominal confluence of lymphatic trunks, is usually located at the level of the 2nd lumbar vertebra. However, there are anatomical variations that might displace the cisterna chyli to be found anywhere between the 10th thoracic vertebra and the 3rd lumbar vertebra. An important anatomical landmark is the cisterna chyli usually located to the right of the abdominal aorta and places the cisterna chyli at risk during abdominal aortic surgery like surgical management of aortic dissection. The cisterna chyli drains both the right and the left lumber trunks as well as the intestinal lymph trunks. The intercostal trunks, however, might enter into the upper part of the cisterna or might empty directly into the thoracic duct. The thoracic duct is the largest lymphatic channel thorough out the body measuring between 38 and 45 mm in length and 2–5 mm in diameter; the length of the duct extends from the 2nd lumbar vertebra superiorly to the base of the neck. It collects the lymph from the entire body except for the right side of the head and neck, hemithorax, and right upper extremity, as these structures drain into the right lymphatic trunk. On a histological level, the thoracic duct is composed of three distinct layers. They are from outer to inner: the adventitia, media, and intima.

Despite the considerable variation in the origination point of the thoracic duct, the most common origination point comes from the superior pole of the cisterna chyli, the thoracic duct then heads north and pass through the diaphragm, then it continues ascending into the inferioposterior section of the mediastinum, the mediastinum contains various anatomic critical structures like the thoracic aorta, azygos and hemiazygos veins where the thoracic duct is sandwiched between the diaphragm and the esophagus anteriorly and the vertebral column and the intercostal arteries posteriorly [4]. The thoracic duct starts taking a left direction at the level of the 5th thoracic vertebra in which it enters the superior mediastinum. It ultimately makes its way into the left neck, where the thoracic duct arches laterally 3–4 cm above the clavicle. This takes place at the level of the 7th cervical vertebra. The duct usually terminates by opening into the junction of the left subclavian and internal jugular veins in 32%; however, variations of this relationship do exist as the duct might open to one of the two veins exclusively: the internal jugular vein in 46% while the subclavian vein in 18% or might divide into several smaller vessels that individually open into the venous system. This area is referred to in as the lympho-venous junction [2, 5]. While the classical anatomical typical course has been described, it has been anticipated that it is present in only 40–60% of patients, often complicating already challenging variable anatomy. There are nine proposed likely variations of the thoracic duct that Davis described in 1915. This description originated subsequent to the dissection of 22 cadavers and looking at which embryonic thoracic duct prevails and which one atrophies, it was found that the most frequent anatomic variation of the thoracic duct is a doubling of the lower part of the duct caused by the persistence of both right and left trunks. In a more extensive series, the incidence of doubling was reported between 39% and 47% [6, 7]. It is advocated that the termination of the thoracic duct into the left great veins of the neck takes place between 92% and 95% and happens on the right side of the neck in 2–3% and bilaterally in 1% of the time. The anatomy of the lymphatic system is more complicated than the description provided in classical anatomical textbooks [5].

Drainage Patterns of Various Anatomic Subsites of the Head and Neck

Understanding the distribution of cervical lymph node metastases of various head and neck cancer subsites helps determine the necessity of level IV dissection. Lindberg's landmark paper in 1972 was designed to serve that purpose – to avoid dissecting lymph node levels not commonly involved by each head and neck subsite and to minimize any morbidity associated with dissecting the levels. He reviewed the records of 2,044 patients with previously untreated squamous cell carcinomas of the head and neck to define the incidence and anatomical distribution of lymph node metastases [8]. He looked at three subsites specific for oral cavity cancer, and they were oral tongue, the floor of the mouth, and retromolar trigone. For oral tongue, level IV was rarely involved [5/169], and level V was involved even less [1/169].

The floor of mouth cancer showed a very similar pattern [6/127 and 1/127, respectively].

Similarly, retromolar trigone involved only 5/170 level IV nodes and 1/170 level V nodes. Based on the decision tree analysis, Weiss et al. recommended elective nodal dissection when the incidence of occult metastases is greater than 20% [9]. When the risk is less than 20%, the morbidity of surgery outweighed the benefit. This threshold is still widely accepted when determining the necessity for elective neck dissection. Thus, under this standard, dissection of levels IV and V would not be indicated for oral cavity cancer.

The paradigm shift from radical neck surgeries to more selective types of neck dissections – most commonly selective neck dissection (I-III)/supraomohyoid neck dissection (SOHND) and their comparable neck control rates in N0 oral cavity cancer – has been described by many authors [10, 11]. However, other authors argued that SOHND is inadequate surgery for oral tongue carcinoma, due to occult skip metastasis to level IV and that level IV should be routinely included in neck dissection for N0 oral tongue cancer [12, 13]. Understandably, this "extended" selective neck dissection for oral tongue carcinoma would significantly increase the risk of chyle leak. However, the concept of extended selective neck dissection to clear skip metastasis has been challenged by recently published articles. Warshavsky et al. performed a systematic review and meta-analysis on the rate of skip metastasis to neck level IV in oral cavity squamous cell carcinoma [14]. This study showed the meager rate of skip metastasis to neck level IV in the clinically negative neck (<5.5%). The study not only showed the overall rate of level IV involvement to be less than 11.4% but also showed that the rate of level IV skip metastasis did not increase significantly in cases that involved neck levels I-III. Based on these findings, removal of level IV is not indicated for N0 neck oral cavity carcinoma, or even when suspicious nodes are encountered in levels I-III intraoperatively during neck dissection. For N0 neck, the only time clearance of level IV is indicated would be when a suspicious node is encountered intraoperatively at level IV. Another recent study from Kobe, Japan [15] looked at 100 oral carcinoma patients with any cTN1M0 stage and found out that level V was never involved. Level IV was involved in only two patients with tongue carcinoma. However, these two cases were not skip metastasis, since both of them were found to have positive nodes in level II as well. The author concluded that level IV dissection should be considered in patients with tongue cancer and clinical lymph-node metastasis at level II. This study considered 45 tongue cancer patients. Thus, 2/45 (4.4%) do not meet the threshold of 20% for the indication of neck dissection in level IV.

In conclusion, regardless of the primary tumor and nodal stage, there is no clear indication to include levels IV-V in neck dissection for oral cavity squamous cell carcinoma. The only indication to include level IV or level V would be clinically or radiographically positive lymph nodes in these levels. Therefore, in light of the risk of chyle leak, dissection of these levels without clear indications cannot be justifiable in oral cancer.

Risk Factors of Chyle Leak

Hypothetically, the thoracic duct is at risk for iatrogenic injury during any transcervical procedures, especially those procedures that require surgical manipulation with lower cervical nodes such as level III and IV cervical lymph groups. Some of the contributing factors that might increase the risk of iatrogenic injury are the inconstant anatomy of the duct as well as its tenuous nature [2]. Likewise, some clinical situations might raise that risk such as lower neck surgery, neck dissection especially if metastatic neck disease is present and is involving level IV, history of previous radiation therapy, particularly if the lower part of the neck was incorporated within the radiation field, and finally surgeon's experience [2, 5]. From a neck dissection perspective, posterolateral neck dissection defined as the dissection of levels (II-V) lymph node groups and lateral neck dissection, which typically harvests lymph nodal groups (II-IV), might be associated with increased risk of chylous leak [16, 17]. This was previously considered as a form of selective neck dissection according to the 1991 classification by the committee of the American Head and Neck Society and the American Academy of Otolaryngology-Head and Neck Surgery [16]. In addition, radical and modified radical neck dissections have a similar increased risk of chyle leak. In general, the risk of chyle leak ensuing from any type of neck dissection ranges between 2% and 8%. Neck ablative procedure other than a neck dissection that might be associated with risk of chyle leak is thyroidectomy especially if it is happening in conjunction with central neck dissection or if level VI nodal group is harbored with metastatic disease and needs to be included in the surgical dissection. Thyroidectomies are associated with a chyle leak risk that ranges between 0.5% and 1.4% [2]. Other causes of chyle leak are nontraumatic in nature such as idiopathic chylous fistulas, mostly reported when malignancies are situated at the lympho-venous junction such as lymphoma. Other causes of nontraumatic chyle leaks are inflammatory, lymphatic malformation, and finally, autoimmune diseases (Table 4.1).

Table 4.1 Risk factors for developing chyle leak

Traumatic/surgically induced:
Traumatic injuries to the lower neck region (MVC, gun-shut wounds to Zone I)
Thoracic surgery (esophagectomy, mediastinal tumors, pneumonectomy)
Cardiac surgery for (patent ductus arteriosus, coarctation of the aorta]
Neck surgery, especially neck dissection and thyroid surgery
Abdominal surgery (Radical lymph node dissection, aortic dissection)
Interventional procedures (left heart catheterization, subclavian vein catheterization)
Nontraumatic:
Idiopathic
Autoimmune (Sarcoidosis, Bechet's disease)
Inflammatory conditions
Other non-head and neck malignancies (lymphoma, metastatic disease]
Lymphatic abnormality (Gorham disease, lymphangiomyomatosis]

The Risk of Lower Neck Nodal Involvement in Head and Neck Cancer

As surgeons who treat metastatic neck disease in the setting of head and neck cancers, it is crucial to differentiate between the management of a neck with no clinical/radiographic features of metastatic disease, commonly referred to as N0 neck and necks with metastatic disease. Occult metastases are defined as tumor metastases to lymph nodes that cannot be detected with clinical exam or radiographic studies. In N0 neck, occult metastases range between 20% and 44%; 40% of total body lymph nodes are located in the head and neck region and contained within the fibro-fatty tissues between the neck musculature. The accuracy of identifying and staging of neck disease is crucial in many phases of care for patients with head and neck cancer. Selecting the appropriate surgical intervention, need for adjuvant therapy, and ultimately overall survival are also pivotal. Selective neck dissection seems to be a proper treatment for patients with N0 disease, especially with a recurrence risk of 5% in the dissected nodal basin or outside the dissected basin, including contralateral nodes; various authors support this. Manni and Van Den Hoogen found a slightly increased percentage but still within the single-digit risk of recurrent neck disease of approximately 7% with oral cavity cancers. This risk of recurrence seemed to be elevated in primary laryngeal and pharyngeal cancers approaching 11% [18]. As any surgical procedure, the operating surgeon's experience continues to play an imperative role in outcomes from a neck dissection.

Complications Arising from Chyle Leak

Understanding the troubling complications that might arise from unaddressed chyle leak explains why the published literature about this topic stresses the need for early identification. These complications include compromised wound healing as chyle leaks tend to cause a disruption in the biochemical environment in the neck, as well as decreasing blood supply to the developed neck skin flaps [2] leading to necrosis (Fig. 4.1) and exposure of the deep neck structures to the open environment. Skin flap necrosis in itself can potentially lead to infections, which compromise other skin tissues, or potentially disseminating to involve different neck subunits or spread into the deeper neck spaces such as the retropharyngeal space and mediastinum (Fig. 4.2). It is the authors' experience that these infections in a previously or freshly dissected necks tend to spread rapidly, and this might be credited to the violation of the neck fascial planes that almost always take place in any neck dissection. The duration of the chyle leak is an important variable when it comes to expecting complications; the more prolonged chylous leaks are left unaddressed, the higher the chances of developing a more chronic cumbersome fistula. Finally, if the volume of chyle leak is high enough to create abundant hydrostatic pressure, it might penetrate through thoracic pleura, forming a

Fig. 4.1 Central skin flap necrosis. Note this is the neck bed after serial debridement, Wound VAC therapy

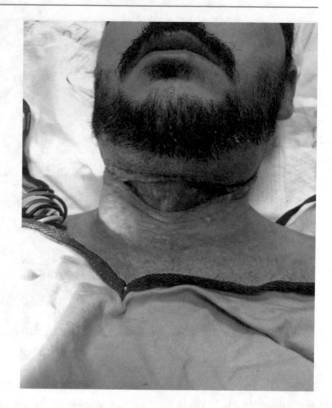

chylothorax. One of the early signs of a chylothorax is patients complain of dyspnea, tachypnea, and chest pain [2]. Another potential complication that might arise from high volume chyle leak would be airway compromise, especially if a surgical airway was not performed (Fig. 4.3).

Diagnosis of Chyle Leak

As a complication arising from a neck dissection, chyle leak diagnosis can take place in two different settings, either intraoperatively or postoperatively. In the intraoperative setting, there are usually two scenarios. First, if the chyle leak was identified during the neck dissection, the surgeon should pause the neck dissection and attempt to control the chylous leak by ligating the thoracic duct. General neck inspection should be a routine step immediately after the completion of neck dissection when the neck is inspected for any bleeding vessels, irrigate the neck, and finally, inspect for any chylous leaks. This is usually presented clinically as white milky fluid (Fig. 4.4). The best location to inspect chyle leak will be the supraclavicular region while retracting the sternocleidomastoid muscle gently laterally. Many reasons might complicate immediate intraoperative identification. The first reason is the variable and inconsistent location and course of the thoracic duct

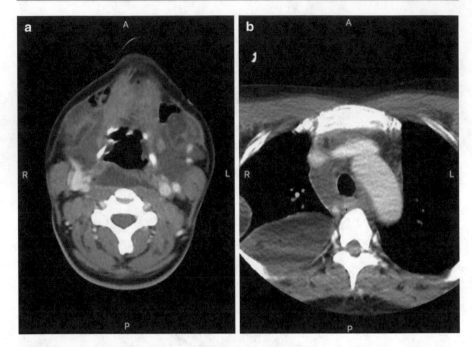

Fig. 4.2 (**a**). Infection spreading into the retropharyngeal space. (**b**). Spread of the infection into the mediastinum

something we eluded to in the anatomy section of this chapter. The second reason is collapsibility of the thoracic duct. Finally, a contributing factor is the NPO status of patients undergoing neck dissection. The combination of these factors might preclude the surgeon from intraoperative chyle leak identification. Experts in the head and neck surgery field recommend the utilization of magnifying surgical loups in an attempt to aid intraoperative identification. There are some maneuvers the surgeon might implement to facilitate chyle leak identification.

Intraoperative Valsalva Maneuver

Historically, the Valsalva maneuver was envisioned by Antonio Maria Valsalva, an Italian anatomist. He performed this maneuver 300 years ago; the primary purpose of this maneuver is to remove foreign bodies and exudates from the middle ear. Originally this maneuver was executed by awake patients by performing an expiratory effort. At the same time, the mouth is closed as well as the glottis in a sitting or supine position for 10–20 s. Usually, this maneuver increases the intra-oral pressure as well as the intrathoracic pressure by 40 mmHg, followed by a sudden pressure release in which normal breathing is restored. This maneuver can also be achieved by forced expiration by contracting the thoracic and abdominal muscles strongly

Fig. 4.3 Significant swelling of the neck bilaterally – a complication of postoperative chyle leak, diagnosed after T2, N2B, M0 (floor of mouth squamous cell carcinoma)

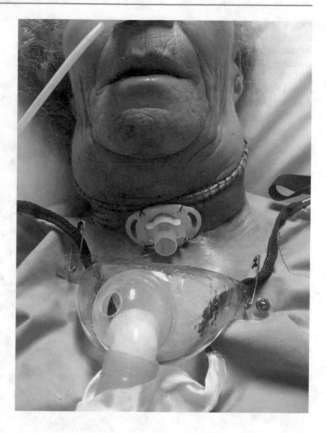

against high airway resistance. Some protective reflexes such as sneezing, gagging, and vomiting can imitate a Valsalva maneuver. In the operating room, the anesthesia team might perform the Valsalva maneuver. At the same time, the patient is asleep by the prevention of expiration, while gas flow continues to enter the circuit with an adjustable pressure valve that is partially or fully closed. The surgeon requesting this maneuver should be aware of the significant physiological ramifications. These changes are beyond the scope of this chapter, but we are going to mention some of them. Valsalva maneuver causes a significant increase in intrathoracic pressure, which activates the aortic arch baroreceptor triggering a decrease in heart rate. Another physiological change occurring from this maneuver is the reduction of the venous return, which manifests itself as distention of the jugular veins. After the release of the airway closure, some physiological compensations take place, namely, the fall in the intrathoracic pressure and pooling of blood in the pulmonary vessels, which causes a transient decrease in the blood pressure.

The Valsalva maneuver can be used to identify chyle leak by increasing the chyle flow and improve visibility as well as any bleeding vessels in the neck. The percentage of successful identification of bleeding points using the Valsalva maneuver reaches 30% [19].

Fig. 4.4 The thoracic duct. Identification intraoperatively of the thoracic duct during dissection of a suspicious level IV lymph node during a left neck dissection

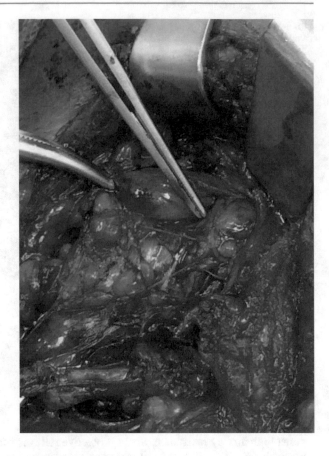

Management of Chyle Leak

Management of chyle leak can be categorized into immediate intraoperative management, conservative medical postoperative management, and postoperative surgical chyle leak management.

Immediate Intraoperative Management

Intraoperative chyle leak starts with attempts to identify the thoracic duct. This might be facilitated with a Valsalva maneuver. If the duct is identified, then attempts should be made to ligate the duct with clips or tying the duct. The authors recommend over suturing the duct while paying great attention to the internal jugular and the subclavian vessels. Local muscular flaps are great in managing chyle leaks.

Identification and Ligation

Prevention and surgical care should be exercised in any neck surgery, mainly when performed on the left side or in levels III and IV. Other than relying on the anatomical exploration to identify the thoracic duct, newer technologies have emerged in head and neck cancer procedures. One of them is Indocyanine Green, which is currently used in various medical procedures, something that has been used in free flap angiography to confirm patency and flow in free flaps microvascular anastomosis. Other uses of this technology is for lymphangiography in various treatment such as surgical treatment of lymphedema, and recently for the identification of the thoracic duct (Table 4.2) [20]. After the thoracic duct is identified, then it should be protected. If an inadvertent injury occurred, then it should be isolated and ligated. Some surgeons advocate the use of hemostatic agents, such as cyanoacrylate adhesives, namely, Dermabond®; fibrin glue such as Baxter TISSEEL® and ECIVEL®; and Polyglactin Vicryl mesh [2].

Local Flaps

One of the most commonly used flaps is the sternocleidomastoid muscle flap (SCM) that is almost always exposed during various types of neck dissections. This muscle has segmental blood supply as the superior 2/3rd of the muscles is supplied with branches from the occipital artery. In contrast, the lower 1/3rd is supplied by the thyrocervical trunk. The SCM motor innervation comes from the accessory nerve, while the sensory arises from the cervical plexus. A superiorly based flap helps augment the clipped, or the over sutured duct. Surgeons should avoid utilizing the SCM muscle in previously radiated head and neck cancer patients because of the increased risk of carotid exposure and the muscle itself atrophies after radiation therapy. Some surgeons do not raise the full SCM flap. Still, they tend to advance the muscle and

Table 4.2 Recommendations, steps to use Indocyanine Green with near-infrared imaging system in identifying the thoracic duct and contraindications

Recommendation:
Left + ve neck disease, with clinical or radiographic signs of level IV involvement
Left + ve neck disease, with bulky neck disease at level III
Identification of active chyle leak that is hard to identify via standard neck exploration
Technique:
After the initiation of the neck dissection, 15–20 min before approaching this risk region in the neck, the dorsum of the left foot is injected subcutaneously with ICG. This step could be performed by the anesthesia team or the non-scrubbed surgical team members. 25 mg of powder ICG is reconstituted in 10 ml of sterile saline to create a 2.5 mg/ml concentration. A 25-gauge needle with a 5 ml syringe is required.
The operative room light should be lowered or turned off completely; the overhead operating table should also be lowered without compromising the neck dissection process and the surgeon's visualization of the surgical field.
1–2 ml are injected before imaging is performed using a handheld near-infrared device that is over draped with a sterile transparent cover, by directing the imaging device toward the junction between the internal jugular vein and the subclavian vein. If the thoracic duct was not identified, the injection could be repeated as needed.
Contraindication and Precautions:
Iodine hypersensitivity
Dialysis, renal failure, uremia
Pregnancy and breastfeeding
Laboratory test interference such as radioactive iodine

suture on top of the ligated thoracic duct [21] (Fig. 4.5). Other local flaps the authors used is the scalene muscle flap again not raised independently but rotated on top of the ligated thoracic duct [2].

Postoperative Diagnosis of Chyle Leak

If all intraoperative maneuvers failed to reveal a leak, a high degree of postoperative suspicion should be exercised, especially when there is an unexplained increase in the drain output, particularly if fat-containing diet or formula is resumed. The clinical exam might show signs of neck erythema or fluid collection [2]. To confirm your clinical diagnosis, the milky fluid should be sent for analysis; the triglyceride levels will be >100 mg/dL along with the presence of chylomicrons (Fig. 4.6).

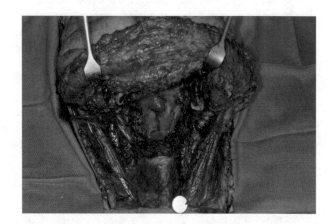

Fig. 4.5 Left SCM muscle mobilized after completion of the neck dissection and advanced to re-enforce the ligated thoracic duct in T4a, N2C, M0 after total glossectomy. Red arrow shows the advancement of the left SCM; the white circle is the location of the ligated thoracic duct

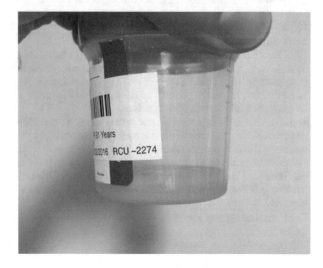

Fig. 4.6 Clinical collection of chyle from the drain, which was later confirmed with elevated triglyceride levels >100 mg/dl as well as the presence of chylomicron

Postoperative Management

Postoperative management of chyle leak could be categorized under medical management arm versus a surgical management arm. If medical management is unsuccessful in decreasing the output from the chyle leak, radiographic interventional options, as well as surgical options, are available.

Conservative Management

Conceptually, conservative management of a chyle leak involves closure by secondary intention: decrease the lymphatic output and obliterate surgical dead space [22]. Several options can be used in conjunction to improve the chances of closure, including activity modification, diet modification, wound care, and pharmacologic options. Most fistulas will resolve with these measures alone; however, this complication will certainly lengthen hospital stay. Notably, more aggressive surgical measures are warranted when fistula persists for more than 14 days. There are surgical complications or metabolic disturbances that might arise. Due to the relative infrequency of this complication, there are no randomized control trials to guide decision-making, instead of case reports, cohort studies, and algorithms based on clinical experience.

Activity Modification

Chyle flow is modulated by physical activity and Valsalva pressure. An initial conservative measure for patients with a suspected leak is bed rest, head of bed elevation (30–40°), and stool softeners to decrease intrathoracic and intra-abdominal pressure during defecation.

Diet Modification

The dietary change serves two objectives: replenishment of losses and slow down flow rate. Chyle loss necessitates the replacement of fluids, electrolytes, and protein. Regardless of parentral or entral delivery, the treating team must match losses to create euvolemia, replace electrolytes judiciously, and support postoperative nutrition.

Medium Chain Triglyceride (MCT)

Diet is typically nonfat, low-fat, or medium-chain triglyceride (MCT). Theoretically, short- and medium-chain fatty acids are water-soluble, absorbed by the portal venous circulation. This mechanism bypasses gastrointestinal lymphatics, and therefore, decreases chyle production at the GI source. However, dietary modification does not stop the flow completely, necessitating a combination approach described throughout this chapter. Moreover, there is controversy in pursuing a modulated fat diet. A study by Benedix et al. demonstrated that while on an MCT and water-only diet, chylomicron and triglycerides can paradoxically increase by 20% in some patients [23]. These types of results introduce the concept of TPN upfront, although generally not standard in most algorithms. Certainly, this underscores the controversy surrounding this topic.

Elemental Formula

For many patients for whom PO intake is contraindicated, enteral feeding with elemental formula is considered. Specifically, for low output leaks, the literature suggests low fat, semi-elemental formula. For higher output leaks, elemental formula should be employed [10]. As nutrition is parsed into its building blocks, clinicians should ensure items such as vitamins (including fat soluble) and minerals are carefully replaced.

Total Parenteral Nutrition (TPN)

Total parenteral nutrition (TPN) is generally applied for high output leaks, or when enteral modification has failed to decrease the output. TPN allows for complete bypass of the gastrointestinal system, thus decreasing chyle production from the source [23, 24]. However, TPN presents classic disadvantages: line infection, bacteremia, and venous thrombosis. While these disadvantages can be mitigated through judicious central line hygiene and prophylactic anticoagulation, the duration of TPN is a risk factor for complications [25].

Wound Care

Suction Drains

Suction drains placed at the time of surgery are the first indicator of chyle fistula, evacuate accumulated fluid, and monitor the flow to evaluate the effectiveness of therapy. While usage of drainage is standard, some clinicians advocate for prompt removal when output diminishes as suction may delay resolution. One study by Dhiwakar et al. notes that removal of drains and serial aspiration lead to the successful resolution of chyle leak for six patients of their series [26, 18].

Pressure Dressings

A supraclavicular pressure dressing is widely used in the initial management of chyle fistula. While advocates recognize an expedited closure, others note a concern with overlying skin flap comprise, as well as free flap compromise if this procedure was utilized for reconstruction [27–29]. Clinicians may use spongy orthopedic foam tape with gauze in the supraclavicular area. The taping pattern varies but is most efficient when applied in multiple vectors, both perpendicular across the chest and superio-inferiorly.

Negative Pressure Wound Therapy

Wound vacuum, also known as negative pressure wound therapy (NPWT), is described through case series. Generally, NPWT allows for the extraction of fluid, decrease of inflammatory mediators, increased oxygen, decreased bacterial counts, and facilitation of granulation tissue. Dorneden et al. provide excellent results when placing the black foam sponge approximately 5 cm away from the chyle fistula, with their vacuum set at 125 mmHg. Moreover, this group describes the placement of white, nonporous polyvinyl alcohol foam to protect the great vessels from subatmospheric suction. Their concept is to close the dead space by using negative pressure to induce the collapse of the thoracic duct [30].

Pharmacological Methods

Somatostatin

Somatostatin (SS) is extensively described in the cardiothoracic surgery literature to treat chylothorax [31]. Also known as growth hormone inhibiting hormone, SS is widely used in endocrinology for acromegaly and neonatal hyperinsulinism, gastroenterology for intractable diarrhea, severe gastrointestinal bleed, and oncology for carcinoid and tumors secreting vasoactive intestinal peptide [32, 33]. In the resolution of cervical chyle leaks, the exact mechanism is unknown, although two considerations have been postulated: vasoconstriction of lymphatic vasculature, or vasoconstriction of splanchnic vessels and decreased intestinal perfusion [34]. Side effects are related to reduced GI mobility: nausea, malabsorption, diarrhea, flatulence, cholelithiasis, and biliary obstruction. More rarely, less than <1% of patients demonstrate anaphylaxis. Octreotide, a synthetic SS analog, is the typical drug delivery, specifically, 100 mcg subcutaneously 2–3 times per day. A 2015 publication by Swanson et al. demonstrates effectiveness in combination with MCD and suction drainage, followed by TPN if output did not resolve. Notably, the 12 patients in their study showed chyle leaks with an average output of 445.5 cc in the previous 24 h before treatment. The results note fistula closure at 5.5 days and decreased length of hospital stay to an average of 8.7 days, with 0/12 patients requiring surgery [35]. Again, this is in comparison to other studies where SS was not utilized; patients had prolonged hospital stays averaging over 30 days, and increased likelihood of significant morbidity requiring surgery.

Orlistat

Orlistat is a pancreatic lipase inhibitor and was described by Belloso et al. in 2006 [36]. In this review, lipase is secreted at the duodenum and breaks down triglycerides to monoglycerides and free fatty acids. These products are combined with cholesterol and phospholipids, and then absorbed as chylomicrons at the jejunum and ileum, thereby forming chyle. Orlistat is typically utilized to treat obesity; for chyle fistula management, lipase inhibition results in dramatically reduced chyle flow. Belloso et al. used a dosing regimen of 120 mg TID, taken 30 min before meals, and noted all four patients had fistulas resolve within 14 days. Of note, side effects include abdominal discomfort, steatorrhea, and fecal urgency; however, these are mitigated by employing a low-fat diet.

Etilefrine

Etilefrine is an alpha- and beta-adrenergic sympathomimetic amine and is detailed in the cardiothoracic literature. Typically utilized for postural hypotension, etilefrine is thought to constrict the smooth muscles of the main lymphatic vessels, thus decrease chyle flow [37, 38]. Guillem et al. [37] utilized the agent for chylothorax or chyloperitoneum in a series of 10 patients with promising results. Their dosing regimen was 4.2–5 mg/h intravenous infusion in addition to conservative measures. The mean treatment duration was 6.4 days, which dropped the daily output from 740 cc to 183 cc. Classic side effects to this medicine include headache, flushing, palpitations, and nervousness. Practitioners should be mindful of patients with cardiomyopathy as this cardioactive agent can lead to increase heart rate and blood pressure. There are no instances of use in the head and neck literature, although etilefrine may warrant further studies.

Invasive and Surgical Treatment

Percutaneous Transabdominal Lymphatic Access

Utilizing fluoroscopic-guided imaging to identify cisterna chyli or retroperitoneal lymphatic duct is accessed transabdominal. Access line is gained with a 21-gauge 20 cm Chiba needle under constant fluoroscopic imaging. A thin guide wire 0.018 is advanced into the Chiba needle and is advanced cephalic toward the thoracic duct. An introducer system is cylindered over the wire after this step is done with iodinated contrast is used to identify and confirm the location of the chyle leak by visualization of extravasation. There are many liquid embolic and coil materials of the interventional radiologist's preference that he/she can use to embolize the thoracic duct and some if its proximal extension (Table 4.3) [39, 40].

It should be noted that lymphatic fluid does not contain coagulation factors and thrombotic factors such as blood, a fact that might make the use of coils to augment liquid embolic materials are realistic mainly that these materials mechanism of action depends on blood contact to polymerize and form the cast [41]. Other less popular agents that might be used are sclerosing agents; however, it should be noted that these agents tend to complicate surgical re-exploration if indicated. Complications to adjacent structures might arise such as phrenic nerve injury [42].

Transcervical Thoracic Duct Puncture

This is indicated for surgical and traumatic chyle leaks near the junction of the internal jugular and the subclavian veins. In this technique, the thoracic duct is identified using a combination of ultrasound guidance to avoid injury to vascular structures as well as fluoroscopy to confirm the location of the thoracic duct. This maneuver is usually started after lymphangiography is performed to locate the thoracic duct and similar to the percutaneous transabdominal lymphatic access similar technique is used.

Surgical Exploration

There are no hard conscience on when these options should be utilized; however, the general recommendation that if the chyle output is between 500 and 1000 ml/day for 5 days or more, especially with lack of any improvement in conservative medical management. Many factors might obscure the identification of the thoracic duct like the local inflammation that occurs locally in the neck from the chyle leak and if previous sclerosing agents were used. However, previously mentioned maneuvers might facilitate the identification of the thoracic duct, which can be ligated or clipped. It is recommended to have multimodality control of the thoracic duct, especially in the case of second surgical exploration. We recommend the use of local flaps, which were mentioned in the immediate intraoperative management of chyle leak.

Table 4.3 Embolization materials used for chyle leak management	
	N-butyl-2-cyanoacrylate/NBCA glue
	Onyx® (ev3, Irvine, California)
	Histoacryl/acrylic glue
	Fibrin Glue Baxter TISSEEL®, ECIVEL®
	Sclerosing agents (OK-432, tetracycline)
	Polyglactin Vicryl mesh
	Coils (metal/steel/mini/Gianturco/GAW)
	Embosphere (BioSphere ® Medical, Merit Medical Systems Inc)
	Microcoil (Tornado® COOK Inc)

Thoracoscopic Ligation of the Thoracic Duct

This is the last resort if all the aforementioned treatments failed to control the output of the chyle leak. Three-port thoracoscopy is used to identify where the location of the thoracic duct between the aorta and azygus vein, and the thoracic duct is clipped with 3–4 clips. In general, this procedure does not require the use of double-lumen intubation. Complications that might arise from this treatment modality include lung injury and potential disruption of other lymphatic branches, which might give rise to chylothorax [43].

Conclusion

Head and neck surgeons performing cervical procedures, especially neck dissections, should be aware of chyle leak as a potential complication that may arise from left neck dissection, especially when level IV lymph nodes are included in the dissection and prevention. Immediate intraoperative management will save the surgeon the exhausting exercise of postoperative management including both arms of conservative medical management and invasive surgical management. Figure 4.7 describes the algorithm of chyle leak management.

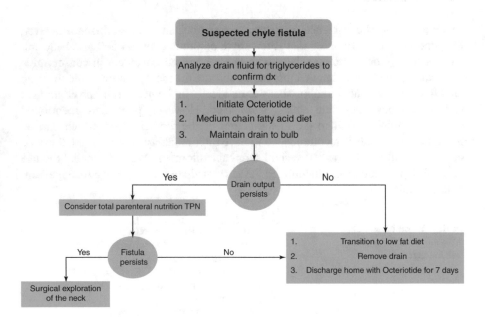

Fig. 4.7 Algorithm adapted from (Delaney et al. [2])

References

1. Johnson OW, Chick JFB, Chauhan NR, Fairchild AH, Fan C-M, Stecker MS, et al. The thoracic duct: clinical importance, anatomic variation, imaging, and embolization. Eur Radiol. 2015;26(8):2482–93.
2. Delaney SW, Shi H, Shokrani A, Sinha UK. Management of Chyle leak after head and neck surgery: review of current treatment strategies. Int J Otolaryngol. 2017;2017:8362874.
3. Abbas AK, Lichtman AH, Pillai S. Cellular and molecular immunology. Philadelphia: Saunders; 2014. 1 p
4. Gilroy AM, MacPherson BR, Ross LM. Atlas of anatomy. New York: Thieme; 2012. 1 p.
5. Smith ME, Riffat F, Jani P. The surgical anatomy and clinical relevance of the neglected right lymphatic duct: review. J Laryngol Otol. 2013;127(2):128–33.
6. Hematti H, Mehran RJ. Anatomy of the thoracic duct. Thorac Surg Clin. 2011;21(2):229–38–ix.
7. Davis HK. A statistical study of the thoracic duct in man. Am J Anat. 1915;17(2):211–44.
8. Lindberg R. Distribution of cervical lymph node metastases from squamous cell carcinoma of the upper respiratory and digestive tracts. Cancer. 1972;29(6):1446–9.
9. Weiss MH, Harrison LB, Isaacs RS. Use of decision analysis in planning a management strategy for the stage N0 neck. Arch Otolaryngol Head Neck Surg. 1994;120(7):699–702.
10. Medina JE, Byers RM. Supraomohyoid neck dissection: rationale, indications, and surgical technique. Head Neck. 1989;11(2):111–22. John Wiley & Sons, Ltd.
11. Fakih AR, Rao RS, Borges AM, Patel AR. Elective versus therapeutic neck dissection in early carcinoma of the oral tongue. Am J Surg. 1989;158(4):309–13.
12. Byers RM, Weber RS, Andrews T, McGill D, Kare R, Wolf P. Frequency and therapeutic implications of "skip metastases" in the neck from squamous carcinoma of the oral tongue. Head Neck. 1997;19(1):14–9. John Wiley & Sons, Ltd.
13. Dias FL, Lima RA, Kligerman J, Farias TP, Soares JRN, Manfro G, et al. Relevance of skip metastases for squamous cell carcinoma of the oral tongue and the floor of the mouth. Otolaryngol Head Neck Surg. 2006;134(3):460–5. SAGE PublicationsSage CA: Los Angeles.
14. Warshavsky A, Rosen R, Nard-Carmel N, Abu-Ghanem S, Oestreicher-Kedem Y, Abergel A, et al. Assessment of the rate of skip metastasis to neck level IV in patients with clinically node-negative neck oral cavity squamous cell carcinoma: a systematic review and meta-analysis. JAMA Otolaryngol Head Neck Surg. 2019;145(6):542–8. American Medical Association.
15. Kakei Y, Komatsu H, Minamikawa T, Hasegawa T, Teshima M, Shinomiya H, et al. Extent of neck dissection for patients with clinical N1 oral cancer. Int J Clin Oncol. 2020;62(4):212–5. 8 ed. Springer Singapore.
16. Coskun HH, Medina JE, Robbins KT, Silver CE, Strojan P, Teymoortash A, et al. Current philosophy in the surgical management of neck metastases for head and neck squamous cell carcinoma. Head Neck. 2014;37(6):915–26. Eisele DW, editor.
17. Suárez C, Rodrigo JP, Robbins KT, Paleri V, Silver CE, Rinaldo A, et al. Superselective neck dissection: rationale, indications, and results. Eur Arch Otorhinolaryngol. 2013;270(11):2815–21.
18. Clayman GL, Head DFAOO. Selective neck dissection of anatomically appropriate levels is as efficacious as modified radical neck dissection for elective treatment of the clinically negative neck in .... jamanetworkcom; 1998.
19. Kumar CM, Van Zundert AAJ. Intraoperative Valsalva maneuver: a narrative review Manœuvre de Valsalva perope'ratoire: une revue narrative. Can J Anesth. 2018;65(5):578–85. Springer US.
20. Chakedis J, Shirley LA, Terando AM, Skoracki R, Phay JE. Identification of the thoracic duct using indocyanine green during cervical lymphadenectomy. Ann Surg Oncol. 2018;25(12):3711–7.

21. McCraw JB, Arnold PG. McCraw and Arnold's atlas of muscle and musculocutaneous flaps. Norfolk: Hampton PressPub Company; 1988. 1 p.
22. Brennan PA, Blythe JN, Herd MK, Habib A, Anand R. The contemporary management of chyle leak following cervical thoracic duct damage. Br J Oral Maxillofac Surg. 2012;50(3):197–201.
23. Benedix F, Schulz H-U, Scheidbach H, Lippert H, Meyer F. Successful conservative treatment of chylothorax following oesophagectomy – a clinical algorithm. S Afr J Surg. 2010;48(3):86–8.
24. Ramos W, Faintuch J. Nutritional management of thoracic duct fistulas. A comparative study of parenteral versus enteral nutrition. JPEN J Parenter Enteral Nutr. 1986;10(5):519–21.
25. Wang FD, Cheng YY, Kung SP, Tsai YM, Liu CY. Risk factors of catheter-related infections in total parenteral nutrition catheterization. Zhonghua Yi Xue Za Zhi [Taipei]. 2001;64(4):223–30.
26. Dhiwakar M, Nambi GI, Ramanikanth TV. Drain removal and aspiration to treat low output chylous fistula. Eur Arch Otorhinolaryngol. 2014;271(3):561–5.
27. de Gier HH, Balm AJ, Bruning PF, Gregor RT, Hilgers FJ. Systematic approach to the treatment of chylous leakage after neck dissection. Head Neck. 1996;18(4):347–51. John Wiley & Sons, Ltd.
28. Lee YS, Nam K-H, Chung WY, Chang H-S, Park CS. Postoperative complications of thyroid cancer in a single center experience. J Korean Med Sci. 2010;25(4):541–5.
29. Lucente FE, Diktaban T, Lawson W, Biller HF. Chyle fistula management. Otolaryngol Head Neck Surg. 1981;89(4):575–8.
30. Dorneden A, Olson G, Boyd N. Negative pressure wound therapy [wound VAC] in the treatment of chylous fistula after neck dissection. Ann Otol Rhinol Laryngol. 2019;128(6):569–74.
31. Buettiker V, Hug MI, Burger R, Baenziger O. Somatostatin: a new therapeutic option for the treatment of chylothorax. Intensive Care Med. 2001;27(6):1083–6. Springer-Verlag.
32. Shi YF, Harris AG, Zhu XF, Deng JY. Clinical and biochemical effects of incremental doses of the long-acting somatostatin analogue SMS 201-995 in ten acromegalic patients. Clin Endocrinol. 1990;32(6):695–705.
33. Jenkins SA. Drug therapy for non-variceal upper gastrointestinal bleeding. Assessment of options. Digestion. 1999;60(Suppl 3):39–49.
34. Rimensberger PC, Müller-Schenker B, Kalangos A, Beghetti M. Treatment of a persistent postoperative chylothorax with somatostatin. Ann Thorac Surg. 1998;66(1):253–4.
35. Swanson MS, Hudson RL, Bhandari N, Sinha UK, Maceri DR, Kokot N. Use of octreotide for the management of Chyle fistula following neck dissection. JAMA Otolaryngol Head Neck Surg. 2015;141(8):723–7. American Medical Association.
36. Belloso A, Saravanan K, de Carpentier J. The community management of chylous fistula using a pancreatic lipase inhibitor [orlistat]. Laryngoscope. 2006;116(10):1934–5.
37. Guillem P, Papachristos I, Peillon C, Triboulet J-P. Etilefrine use in the management of postoperative chyle leaks in thoracic surgery. Interact Cardiovasc Thorac Surg. 2004;3(1):156–60.
38. Ohkura Y, Ueno M, Iizuka T, Haruta S, Tanaka T, Udagawa H. New combined medical treatment with etilefrine and octreotide for chylothorax after esophagectomy: a case report and review of the literature. Medicine. 2015;94(49):e2214.
39. Itkin M, Kucharczuk JC, Kwak A, Trerotola SO, Kaiser LR. Nonoperative thoracic duct embolization for traumatic thoracic duct leak: experience in 109 patients. J Thorac Cardiovasc Surg. 2010;139(3):584–89–discussion589–90.
40. Toliyat M, Singh K, Sibley RC, Chamarthy M, Kalva SP, Pillai AK. Interventional radiology in the management of thoracic duct injuries: Anatomy, techniques and results. Clin Imaging. 2017;42:183–192. https://doi.org/10.1016/j.clinimag.2016.12.012. Epub 2017 Jan 3. PMID: 28103513.
41. Richter GT, Suen JY. Head and neck vascular anomalies. San Diego: Plural Publishing; 2015. 1 p.
42. Kirse DJ, Suen JY, Stern SJ. Phrenic nerve paralysis after doxycycline sclerotherapy for chylous fistula. Otolaryngol Head Neck Surg. 1997;116(6):680–3.
43. Wilkerson PM, Haque A, Pitkin L, Soon Y. Thoracoscopic ligation of the thoracic duct complex in the treatment for high-volume chyle leak following modified radical neck dissection: safe, feasible, but underutilised. Clin Otolaryngol. 2014;39(1):73–4.

Vascular Complications

5

Anastasiya Quimby, Yoram Fleissig, and Rui Fernandes

Introduction

Neck dissection is intimately involved with rich vasculature of cervical region. Vascular complications in head and neck surgery are rare, but their occurrence requiring intervention indicates poor survival [1]. Patients undergoing elective neck dissections with no prior history of radiation are largely spared from serious complications. Patients with advanced head and neck cancer presenting with bulky nodal disease and requiring chemoradiation therapy are at a higher risk of developing life-threatening vascular complications. The overall incidence and severity of vascular complications have been decreasing over the past decades [2]. This trend is attributed to wide acceptance of selective neck dissection as mainstay of treatment, and improvement in technique with utilization of electrosurgery and diathermy tools [2]. Patient management aimed at the prevention of untoward vascular events is important in reducing morbidity and mortality. Recognition of patients at risk and early intervention are essential in the preventative approach.

This chapter outlines preoperative vascular considerations, possible intraoperative, immediate postoperative and delayed complications, and their management. Additionally, vascular considerations to be taken into account in a setting of microvascular surgery with concomitant neck dissection are described.

A. Quimby (✉) · Y. Fleissig · R. Fernandes
Department of Oral and Maxillofacial Surgery, Division of Head and Neck Oncologic and Microvascular Surgery, University of Florida, Jacksonville, FL, USA
e-mail: rui.fernandes@jax.ufl.edu

© Springer Nature Switzerland AG 2021
T. Schlieve, W. Zaid (eds.), *Complications in Neck Dissection*,
https://doi.org/10.1007/978-3-030-62739-3_5

Preoperative Considerations

Mitigation of intraoperative vascular problems begins with preoperative evaluation of patient's diagnostic imaging. Computed tomography (CT) and, occasionally, magnetic resonance imaging (MRI) scans with intravenous contrast are ordered as part of a standard diagnostic work-up for head and neck cancer patients. These images provide useful information about the extent of nodal disease as well as patient-specific vascular anatomy, presence of any aberrations, and extent of vessel encasement by the tumor mass if present. The decision on whether the risks of morbidity and mortality outweigh the risk of no surgical intervention is made based on an individual basis taking into account several factors. With respect to internal jugular (IJ) vein, a safe distance from the skull base and thoracic inlet to the tumor must be maintained to allow for safe vein ligation. Achieving control of a bleed from the IJ retracted intracranially or into the thorax is exceedingly challenging if not impossible. Tumor encasement of the common or the internal carotid (IC) greater than 270° renders patient a poor surgical candidate due to risks of intraoperative bleeding, stroke, and mortality [Fig. 5.1] [1]. It is important to note that carotid blowout syndrome (CBS) was rarely seen in a patient whose carotid arteries were <180° encased by tumor [3–5].

Preoperative vascular interventions including balloon occlusion testing (BOT), destructive (embolization) or reconstructive (stenting) interventional neuroradiology techniques, and vascular bypass can be considered. Surgeons in 1940s–1960s utilized invasive and noninvasive methods of assessment of circle of Willis in patients with advanced disease. "Matas test" involved application of digital pressure to the carotid and monitoring the patient for immediate changes in mental status [6].

Fig. 5.1 Right neck tumor obliterating the greater vessels

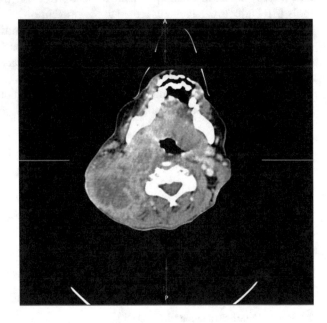

"Dandy's procedure" involved exposure of internal carotid under local anesthetic and temporary complete occlusion of the artery, again monitoring the awake patient for changes in status [7]. BOT involves temporary occlusion of the ipsilateral internal carotid with a nondetachable balloon introduced via femoral artery and assessment for neurologic changes [8]. Although BOT serves as an indicator of risk of acute neurological deficit, some studies have reported development of delayed cerebral ischemia following permanent internal carotid occlusion even in a patient who passed BOT [9]. Nonetheless, carotid embolization is advocated for those high-risk patients who tolerated the test with no neurological impairment. Patients who do not tolerate BOT may be candidates to undergo carotid stenting. Markiewicz et al. described five patients with greater than 270-degree carotid tumor encasement who underwent preoperative stenting of cervical internal or common carotid arteries [10]. In their series, one patient had stent occlusion, which resulted in temporary visual loss and syncopal episodes with no permanent neurologic sequelae [10]. Preoperative stenting afforded adequate oncologic margin resection, and no instances of carotid blowout were recorded during the follow-up period [10]. Carotid bypass surgery with saphenous vein grafts as a definitive option is also mentioned in the literature, despite reports of acceptable rates of postoperative complications. Due to generally poor patient prognosis for patients requiring vascular interventions, no consensus on its applicability exists [1, 11–13].

Surgical techniques were greatly improved in the past decades and some modifications that were adopted specifically aimed to reduce the risk of postoperative vascular complications. Avoiding the placement of a vertical limb of cervical incision along the course of the great vessels was one of the earliest and widely adopted modifications, which was recommended by Shumrick in 1973 [14]. Apron incision reduces the risk of wound break down over the great vessels; this approach was identified as the preferred incision particularly in patients with history of radiation [15]. Classic radical neck dissection as described by Crile not only results in stripping of carotid adventitia, which is a major source of vessel wall nutrition, it also removes the muscle thus leaving it with minimal coverage, which renders the carotid susceptible to CBS [16–18]. Although any neck dissection involves removal of carotid adventitia, the risk of CBS with radical neck dissection was found to be eightfold when compared to selective neck dissection [19].

Intraoperative Vascular Complications

In most instances, when bleeding is encountered intraoperatively, it can be successfully managed with precise use of the monopolar, bipolar electrocautery, suture ties, or hemoclips. Immediate identification of a bleeding vessel is easier to accomplish in a surgical bed that has not been stained with blood from minor bleeds. Keeping surgical field clean also allows for effective control of hemorrhage by allowing for identification, ligation, and division of vessels before they bleed [Fig. 5.2]. When a minor troublesome bleed is difficult to identify after irrigation of surgical bed, requesting the anesthesiologist to perform a Valsalva maneuver and flooding the site

Fig. 5.2 Well-visualized anatomy in a bloodless surgical field

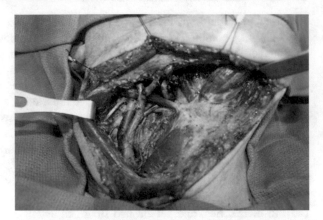

Fig. 5.3 Constant stream of normal saline and suctioning allow for visualization of small bleeding sources within the body of water

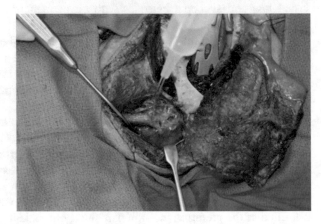

with saline makes even the minor bleeds visible in the body of water and thus manageable (Fig. 5.3). At the conclusion of neck dissection, a thorough inspection of the entire surgical bed and especially levels Ia, IIb, and IV should be completed. Due to their propensity for containing abundant small vessels that may cause postoperative hematoma, placement of thrombin hemostatic agents in those areas can be considered a prophylactic measure.

Difficulty controlling intraoperative hemorrhage arises when the source of bleeding is difficult to access, such as at the skull base or thoracic inlet. Therefore, when IJ ligation is undertaken, it is imperative to ensure that there is a span of vessel available for ligation without risk of retraction into the skull base or thorax while allowing for oncologically sound resection [20]. In the event of IJ bleeding at the skull base, mandibulotomy may be needed for access. Additionally, a short or retracted venous stump may prevent venous walls from collapsing, thus posing a risk for air embolus and a massive bleed requiring immediate action. Due to risk of injury to cranial nerves and other important structures at the cranial base, the urge to blindly hemoclip or ligate should be resisted. Temporizing measures with soaked gauze packing or Fogarty catheter placement maybe employed to slow down the hemorrhage and allow for exploration in a more controlled setting or patient transport to interventional radiology suit for venous embolization [21–23]. Although no reports of jugular bulb or IJ embolization were found in the literature pertaining to neck dissection, a few successful embolizations were reported in trauma and ENT literature and should be considered as an option if surgical exploration fails to establish hemorrhage control [23–25]. Loss of control of distal IJ and its retraction into thoracic cavity is a devastating event that maybe rapidly fatal. Although cervical access can be adequate, in order to improve visualization and ability to gain control, an urgent median sternotomy or clavicle sectioning may be required [22, 26]. As efforts to gain optimal access ensue, attempts to tamponade the bleed with gauze and Fogarty catheter should be made. Anesthesia team must be alerted, and blood transfusion should be initiated as soon as possible since significant amount of blood loss can be expected.

If air entrapment was observed, the surgeon should immediately pack the wound with saline-soaked gauze to prevent further air entry. Next, perform Durant's maneuver, placing the patient in left lateral decubitus position, which will prevent embolus migration to the lungs and allow air to stay in the right heart until resorbed and place the patient in Trendelenburg position to embolus migration into cerebral vasculature and prevent a stroke [21, 27]. Sudden hypotension, decreased end-tidal CO2, and oxygen desaturation can be seen with air embolus [21].

Intraoperative carotid injury, although exceedingly rare, carries high risk of neurological morbidity and mortality. If bleeding from branches of external carotid is difficult to identify and control of a specific branch is not attainable, ligation of external carotid should be done without hesitation and before significant blood loss occurs. It is important to identify at least one branch from the main trunk to ensure that the vessel to be ligated is in fact the external carotid. A large right-angle clamp can be used control hemorrhage and allow for suture ligation and oversewing. Ligation of common or internal carotid should be avoided unless life-threatening hemorrhage occurs.

Early Postoperative Complications

In the immediate postoperative period, hematoma is the most likely complication that can be encountered. In a setting of compromised wound healing, postoperative infection or fistula formation blowout of the great vessels may occur.

By virtue of neck being a highly vascular surgical field, neck surgery is considered a high bleeding risk procedure [28, 29]. Experienced surgeons are well aware of the potential risks of airway compromise, flap compromise, and postoperative infection with hematomas. Nonetheless, the literature pertaining to cervical hematomas occurring after major head and neck surgery is scarce [30]. The reported incidence of hematoma following head and neck procedures ranges from 1% to 5% excluding microvascular surgeries [28, 31]. Occurrence of postoperative hematoma in patients undergoing free tissue transfer is significantly higher and ranges from 11.4% to 30% [30, 32, 33].

Shah-Becker et al. identified male sex, black race, four or more comorbidities, or presence of preoperative coagulopathy as statistically significant risk factors associated with postoperative hematoma in the largest study to date [30]. Of note, they did not find increased incidence of hematoma in patients on anticoagulative and antiplatelet therapy; moreover, they noted that those patients had lower risk of inpatient mortality [30]. Other studies have found that NSAIDs place patients at a significantly higher risk of postoperative hematoma [32]. Preoperatively, safe discontinuation of anticoagulative and antiplatelet therapy is recommended after careful consideration of risks of thromboembolic event versus bleeding. Depending on the therapeutic agent, it may be stopped from 4 to 5 days prior to surgery, like in case of warfarin, or up to hours before surgery with newer agents and heparins [28]. Most current literature recommends restarting anticoagulative and antiplatelet agents within 24–72 h after surgery [28].

Postoperative hematoma that is not a result of carotid or jugular blowout presents within the first few days after surgery as increase in neck swelling, increased sanguineous drain output, and subjective neck tightness. Slow hematoma evolution most likely results from muscle or minor venous channel oozing. Expanding hematomas are not frequently described in association with neck dissections but would present with a sudden onset, rapidly increasing swelling in the neck. Expanding hematoma poses a risk of airway obstruction and significant blood loss, thus should be managed in a timely manner with patient taken back to the operating room for neck exploration. Prior to operating room, cutting of several sutures along the incision line to reduce airway pressure and application of external pressure are useful maneuvers to prevent airway embarrassment and slow down bleeding.

Hematomas have long been thought of as a nidus for infection; thus, operative intervention consisting of hematoma evacuation and neck irrigation is recommended [30, 32]. No consensus regarding prophylactic antibiotic regimen for patients with postoperative hematoma exists. At our institution, antibiotics are given to those patients exhibiting signs or symptoms of infection.

Although a variety of intraoperative hemostatic agents and new methods of electrosurgery are now widely available and utilized, their impact on rates of postoperative hematomas following neck dissections specifically has either not been evaluated or showed no significant difference [34–36].

Nonetheless, meticulous surgical technique with monopolar and bipolar cautery, ultrasonic harmonic scalpels, bipolar LigaSure clamps, appropriate vessel ligation with sutures and/or hemoclips, and application of hemostatic agents into the wound bed should all be employed as deemed appropriate by the surgeon. Occurrence of postoperative hematoma results in increased incidence of wound complications, 540% increased odds of inpatient mortality, increased hospital length of stay, and cost of index admission [30]. The operating surgeon should take all the necessary steps and precautions aimed at reducing the likelihood of postoperative hematoma.

Carotid Blowout Syndrome

Carotid blowout syndrome has long been regarded as one of the most serious and dreaded complications in head and neck surgery. Failure of a weakened arterial wall to withstand intravascular pressure results in vascular rupture [18]. First mentions of the carotid rupture in English language literature date back to 1950s–1960s. In 1959, Mccall reported on four cases of overt common carotid hemorrhage requiring vessel ligation that led to no postoperative neurologic sequalae [6]. Borsanyi commented on the factors associated with carotid rupture and proposed improvements in surgical technique to reduce the likelihood of carotid compromise as well as management of compromised carotid in 1963 [37]. King, in his 1965 article, made mention of carotid rupture as one of the most devastating complications in irradiated patients undergoing head and neck surgery and provided recommendations on skin flap design to minimize the risk of carotid exposure [38]. Although these authors' take on morbidity and mortality associated with the carotid hemorrhage varied, all of them recognized the importance of immediate recognition and prompt management.

In today's literature, carotid artery blowout implies rupture of the extracranial carotid or one of its major branches [39]. More recently, the terminology evolved to recognize carotid blowout syndrome (CBS), which refers to a range of presentations and has been divided into three types: threatened, impending, and acute [13, 39–42]. Type I, threatened CBS, signifies exposure of the carotid either on direct clinical examination or radiographic evidence of tumor invasion of the carotid, pseudoaneurysm, or evidence of air or abscess along the carotid [Fig. 5.4]. In type I CBS there has been no bleeding, but it is expected if no intervention is undertaken. Type II, or impending CBS, refers to occurrence of a self-limiting or easily controlled sentinel

Fig. 5.4 Type 1 CBS due to finding of air pocket in contact with the right common carotid artery (red arrow)

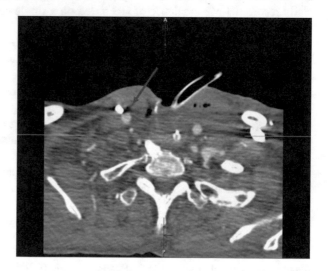

bleed. If no intervention is undertaken, it is certain to evolve into type III over a short period of time. Type III, the acute carotid blowout, is the frank hemorrhage from the extracranial carotid or one of its branches as described by the earlier authors. Recurrent CBS is described as recurrent self-limiting or uncontrollable hemorrhage from the same segment of the arterial wall that underwent treatment a few hours to days after the said treatment, which Suarez et al. consider treatment failure [41, 43]. On the contrary, hemorrhage from a different site along the carotid system that occurs any time after management of previous CBS is considered recurrent CBS due to disease progression [41, 43].

The overall incidence of CBS in patients with head and neck cancer varies from 2.9% to 4.3%. In those undergoing surgical treatment alone, the rate of CBS is 0–2.4%, and in patients with history of previous radiation, the incidence ranges from 4.5% to 21.2% [14, 16, 17, 19, 44–46]. The incidence of CBS in patients with recurrent tumors who underwent reirradiation was reported 0–17% [41].

Internal Jugular Vein Blowout

Not surprisingly, first reports of internal jugular blowout (IJB) appeared in English literature in 1980s as modified radical neck and functional neck dissections gained widespread popularity [47, 48]. IJB is a rare complication with only a few case series reported to date. Presentation of IJB differs from CBS in its severity and symptomology. Acute CBS is likely to be preceded by a single sentinel bleed, whereas acute IJB is heralded by almost daily recurrent self-limiting bleeding episodes that are easily controlled with pressure application [47]. Unlike acute CBS, which if often described as catastrophic or massive bleed, IJ rupture, although may result in life-threatening hemorrhage, clinically appears less severe [49]. Only one study reported 1.3% incidence of IJB based on a single center study, and no other data exists due to a limited number of reports [47].

Predisposing factors for early postoperative vessel blowout are those interfering with wound healing. Specific risk factors are relatively well studied and characterized for CBS but are also believed to contribute to the development of IJB.

At a systemic level, patients with poor nutritional status as demonstrated by rapid weight loss, cachexia, and low albumin have been recognized as high risk for vascular complications early on due to issues with healing [14, 18, 19, 45–50]. In a study that enrolled 102 subjects, Chen at el. demonstrated that patients with BMI <22.5 kg/m^2 ($p < 0.001$) had a twofold increased risk of CBS [19]. Although albumin is a negative acute-phase protein and serves as a poor marker of malnutrition in nonsurgical patients, it was found to be a better predictor of malnutrition than BMI in those undergoing cardiac and orthopedic surgery [51]. Malnutrition and chronic inflammatory states both contribute to poor wound healing. Lu at el. evaluated serum albumin levels in 103 patients with CBS and found that those patients with levels <3.5 g/dL ($p = 0.023$) were more likely to suffer major hemorrhage, and it was an independent predictor of CBS-related death (HR, 3.084:95% CI, 1.267–7.510) [52]. Diabetes mellitus was also named by some authors as a risk factor for CBS, while others saw no statistically significant difference in CBS occurrence in their cohorts [19, 46, 50]. Chronic steroid use, smoking, and alcohol have all been implicated in poor wound healing [17, 48].

With regard to tumor site, oropharyngeal, hypopharyngeal, and laryngeal cancers were more often associated with CBS than other locations [40, 46, 53]. IJB is strongly associated with tumors of larynx and hypopharynx [47, 48, 49].

Radiation therapy, either primary, adjuvant, or reirradiation, has been recognized as one of the most important predisposing factors in the development of CBS [6, 13, 14, 18, 38, 40, 42, 46, 50, 53–57]. Chen et al. found that patients who received radiation dose equal to or greater than 70 Gy had a 12-fold increased risk of CBS [19]. Additionally, reirradiation was associated with a fourfold increased risk of CBS, as well as higher morbidity and mortality rates [41], [46]. Cumulative dose in excess of 130 Gy was associated with a higher risk of CBS as well as other acute and delayed radiation toxicities [41].

Contrary to the conclusive evidence with regard to role of radiation therapy in the development of CBS, there is lack of such convincing evidence when IJB is discussed. It is important to distinguish between the two different types of radiation effects that lead to vascular complications. Early postoperative CBS and IJB develop as a result of poor wound healing imparted by previous radiation injury to the surrounding soft tissues and not as a result of radiation-induced vessel injury. In fact, presence of oro- or pharyngocutaneous fistula has been described in every reported case of IJB, and it further supports the notion that vascular injury is a result of compromised wound healing rather than direct vascular damage. Radiation-injured soft tissues are known to be prone to wound dehiscence, flap necrosis, infections, and oro- or pharyngocutaneous fistula formation with persistent salivary contamination, and all these have been strongly associated with the development of both CBS and IJB [6, 13, 14, 18, 40, 41, 43, 47–49].

Pathophysiology of Early CBS and IJB

In a setting of infection, microemboli formation within vasa vasorum of arteries and localized inflammatory response may result in partial wall necrosis. Similarly, histopathologic studies have demonstrated development of acute phlebitis and venous wall disruption adjacent to abscess formation [47]. Fistula formation results in salivary contamination, which causes enzymatic breakdown of vessel walls leading to eventual vessel rupture [47–49]. Finally, vessel exposure to outside environment because of wound break down leads to its desiccation and failure to maintain its integrity [49].

Presentation and Management

Importance of early recognition and aggressive management cannot be overemphasized.

Wound break down, depending on its extent, can be managed with daily or BID bedside washouts and wet to dry dressing packing. If these measures are not successful, free tissue transfer for wound coverage should be considered promptly [49]. If a surgical site infection is noted, obtaining cultures for targeted antibiotic therapy as well as irrigation and drainage in OR may facilitate earlier resolution of the infection. Management of ora- or pharyngocutaneous fistula may be conservative with wound packing, bedside irrigation, and antisialogogues or may require free tissue transfer. Assessment of the fistula extent can be done with a swallow study utilizing a water-soluble contrast material, gastrografin. Observation of a substantial contrast extravasation should prompt consideration for surgical repair or fistula diversion. Optimization of patient nutritional status should also be prioritized. At times, even with all the appropriate measures taken, patients do progress to IJB and CBS type II or III.

IJB occurs days to weeks following multiple recurrent self-limiting bleeds in a patient with compromised wound healing. Utilization of imaging modalities is questionable since postoperative CT scans are of limited value in the evaluation of small venous bleeds due to the presence of expected postoperative air and fluid in the surgical bed. Thus, diagnosis of IJB relies on the clinical identification of a compromised vessel wall and confirmed by resolution of hemorrhage with IJ ligation. Management of IJB is straightforward in most instances and consists of exploration and IJ ligation away from the area of compromised wall. Suture ligation, oversewing, or adjacent muscle coverage can all be used to ensure control of the proximal and distal venous stumps.

More than 60% of patients present with type III CBS, 25–50% present with impending CBS, and in less than 25% of patients threatened CBS is recognized [13, 40].

In the early postoperative period, days to weeks, type II or type III CBS may present as a self-limiting episode or massive hemorrhage intraorally, in hypopharynx, or as an expanding hematoma and bleeding though incision sites. Obtaining imaging in a setting of type III CBS is virtually impossible due to ongoing or impending patient instability. Centers with immediate interventional radiology capabilities diagnose acute CBS when active extravasation is identified on angiogram in a setting where endovascular management of the lesion is anticipated. Angiography is considered a gold standard for diagnosis of CBS. Chang et al. introduced vascular lesion grading system, which they found to correlate well with clinical types of CBS, and recommended its use to guide management method [58]. Multiple imaging modalities in support of type II CBS diagnosis can be utilized. Vascular lesions noted on computed tomography angiography (CTA), magnetic resonance imaging (MRI), and angiography may range from intravascular irregularity, luminal stenosis, intimal tear to pseudoaneurysm, and frank extravasation [40, 41]. These findings in conjunction with history of a recent self-limiting hemorrhage warrant the diagnosis of impending CBS. The diagnosis of threatened or type I CBS is made in an asymptomatic patient when vessel exposure is observed on clinical examination or noted on a CT or MRI scan. Imaging features consistent with type I CBS include the same as in type II, but with no prior history of bleeding, as well as air, abscess, tumor, or fistula in contact with vessels walls [41]. It is fair to anticipate that with computed tomography being widely available, there will be a shift to higher rates of diagnosis of type I CBS.

Late Postoperative Complications

The most significant delayed vascular complication is CBS that develops years after radiation therapy. Not surprisingly, CBS is more often seen in patients with advanced and recurrent head and neck cancers [3, 9, 13, 46].

Radiation treatment induces free radical formation that causes vasa vasorum microemboli and destruction, adventitial fibrosis, and atherosclerotic changes that progress with time [39, 40, 41, 56, 59]. Murros stipulated that large diameter vessels take proportionately more time to manifest radiation-induced changes [56]. Additionally, radiation-induced localized wall ischemia may lead to pseudoaneurysm formation over the years [45, 60]. Since many patients undergo radiation therapy in conjunction with chemotherapy, it also has been considered as one of the risk factors for CBS [18, 46]. Interestingly, an experimental study carried out by Mittal, to evaluate effects of radiotherapy on the major vessels of canines, did not identify any histopathologic changes suggestive of radiation damage to IJ [61].

Management and Outcomes

Due to high morbidity and mortality, the focus should be on risk assessment and preventative measures to reduce the likelihood of CBS. In high-risk patients undergoing salvage surgery, consideration should be given to soft tissue coverage of cervical carotid with tissue transfer from nonirradiated field [39, 62].

Acute CBS can be rapidly fatal; thus, it requires immediate, systematic, and multidisciplinary intervention. When one encounters acute CBS, presentation can be quite dramatic; therefore, maintaining composure and calm approach to management can be a life-saving step. Similar to acute trauma patient, evaluation and management should focus on airway, breathing, and circulation. Continuous vitals and oxygenation monitoring are of paramount importance as patient status can change rapidly. Immediate and precise pressure application to the cervical portion of the common carotid is more effective at slowing down the hemorrhage than a nontargeted wound packing or generalized neck pressure application. The pulsation of the artery should be palpated, and its trunk should be pinched between the trachea and vertebral column, thus serving as a temporary measure to slow down the hemorrhage. Blood transfusion is very likely; thus orders for blood products should be placed with no delay or STAT (common medical term) this designates that its an emergency order for the staff to prioritize it over any other tasks. In hemodynamically stable patients with a rate of hemorrhage that can be controlled with external maneuvers and no immediate hemodynamic instability is anticipated, endovascular management in hospitals where interventional neuroradiology is immediately available is the preferred initial management [40, 55, 58, 63]. Reconstructive endovascular approach involves deployment of a stent that spans beyond the length of the defect and maintains the blood flow, whereas deconstructive methods involve artery embolization [55, 63]. Occlusion of internal carotid with a detachable balloon in a patient with history of total laryngectomy, right radical neck dissection, and adjuvant radiotherapy with no neurologic sequelae at discharge was first reported in 1984 [64]. Since then, endovascular management gained popularity due to lower rates of morbidity, 10–20% with neurologic sequelae, and mortality </~20%, as compared to artery ligation with 60% and 40%, respectively [14, 16, 19, 41, 45, 50, 55, 65]. Some authors consider emergent endovascular management the only preferred treatment option for acute CBS [9]. Generally, it is preferred to stent internal and common carotid arteries and embolize terminal branches and external carotid artery. Embolization of internal and common carotids is an acceptable option in patients who passed BOT. Although endovascular stenting may offer a better neurologic prognosis, due to concerns for high rate of recurrent bleeding, and stent exposure in a setting of infected or cancerous field, it may not be a suitable definitive management option, but may serve as an acceptable temporizing measure [63], [66]. However, most agree that endovascular embolization, ideally in a patient who is hemodynamically stable enough to pass BOT, is the best approach to management of acute CBS [9, 40, 41].

Surgical intervention for acute CBS is aimed at identification of the source of bleeding and its ligation. Patients with vasculature that has been compromised by significant tumor encasement or any other insult that renders vessel walls too friable and not amenable to surgical manipulation and ligation are at a high risk of intraoperative mortality. They should be counseled preoperatively, and appropriate palliative measures should be undertaken.

When patients are taken to the operating room, special attention must be paid to the maintenance of blood pressure. Hypotension is a well-established factor leading to worse neurologic sequalae [41]. Not infrequently patients with acute CBS are those who recently underwent salvage neck dissection and free tissue transfer; therefore, attempts should be made at preserving vascular pedicle to the flap if at all possible. Once neck is accessed, often times through a recent incision, the surgeon is faced with large clots that must be quickly and efficiently washed out to allow surgical field visualization. Direct common carotid digital pressure can be temporarily applied to slow down the hemorrhage and thus facilitate surgical bed cleaning. Vascular defect maybe readily apparent in a setting of ongoing hemorrhage or may require a Valsalva maneuver to facilitate identification. Rapid cervical carotid artery dissection for circumferential access, clamping, ligation, and oversewing are the only remaining options if patient experiences massive bleeding. Bleeding from terminal branches can be managed with hemoclips, or suture ligation with no concern for neurologic sequalae. If hemorrhage was a result of a small vessel wall defect, the decision should be made if the vessel wall status is amenable to repair rather than complete ligation. Other clotting and hemostatic agents, such as Surgiflo, can be used in the surgical field to facilitate the repairs.

Despite best efforts and most appropriate timely treatment, recurrent bleeding, stroke, and mortality are not uncommon and are likely a result of advanced disease and overall poor patient status rather than vascular event per se [9, 13, 40, 46, 53, 55].

In conclusion, CBS is a heterogeneous range of conditions that may present as an asymptomatic clinical exam or imaging finding or a massive hemorrhage during immediate postoperative period or years after initial surgical intervention. The most important measures a head and neck surgeon can take consist of prompt recognition of high-risk patients and prevention by taking surgical steps to mitigate those risks, such as nonirradiated tissue transfer when applicable.

Vascular Considerations Related to Free Flaps with Concomitant Neck Dissection

Cervical region with its rich blood supply allows for ligation of numerous arteries and veins during a routine neck dissection with no significant sequalae for patients. However, when a free flap reconstruction is planned, care must be taken to ensure that adequate recipient vessels will be available for the microvascular anastomoses.

Performing an elective neck dissection on a neck that has not been previously irradiated or operated on renders vessels easy to identify and preserve. At our institution, we routinely preserve external jugular vein and its branches, if feasible, then identify facial artery and vein at the inferior mandibular border, ligate, divide it, and dissect it off of submandibular gland, thus allowing for a long leash available for anastomosis. We ligate the vessels with hemoclips, thus avoid suture ligation and potential twisting of the vessels on themselves, as well as preserve length. The vessels are kept moist by intermittent irrigation with papaverine and warm saline to prevent vasospasm. Adventitia is known to be a major nutrient supply to vessel walls; thus, adventitial stripping is limited to a short span of the vessel adjacent to the anastomosis. Overzealous vessel preparation may weaken them and make them more susceptible to infectious and enzymatic break down. It is valuable to get into a habit of gentle vessel manipulation and setting them aside in level IB after submandibular gland was removed or medial to sternocleidomastoid soaked in papaverine while the remainder of the neck dissection continues. In this manner, the recipient vessels are protected from inadvertent crush injury by a retractor or hand placement when other neck levels are being addressed.

Neck dissection on a patient, who has been previously irradiated and/or operated on, calls for a much more scrupulous approach. Ablative and reconstructive surgeon must agree on the final surgical plan to ensure that flap design is suitable for a vessel-depleted neck. When possible, flap design should allow for anastomosis to be planned for the side that was not operated on or radiated previously. If that is not an option, several factors must be considered. First, ligated branches of external carotid and both internal and external jugular veins should be anticipated. Thus, alternative recipient vessels must be sought out. Contralateral facial vessels, superior thyroid artery, transverse cervical and internal mammary vessels, and cephalic vein have all been reported as suitable recipient vessels [67, 68]. Additionally, vein grafting can be done in cases where vessel lengths are inadequate. Second, when ipsilateral intact branches exist, their suitability should be assessed. Due to previous surgical and radiation insults, the vessels may be present but have compromised walls that are thickened, calcified, and atherosclerotic or otherwise not suitable for a microvascular anastomosis. Anastomosing a compromised vessel may lead to plaque

Fig. 5.5 Recipient vein was cut back proximally (yellow arrow) to avoid compromised lumen in a setting of a long pedicle

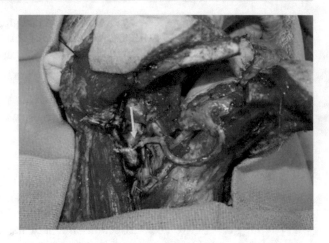

disruption, intraluminal thrombus formation, inability to maintain suture material, or susceptibility to bleeding after surgical manipulation. Additionally, blood flow maybe compromised and result in inadequate flap perfusion. If length of the available pedicle allows, the recipient vessels can be cut back proximally to re-assess for improved blood flow closer to the main trunk [Fig. 5.5].

As a rule of thumb, an ablative surgeon should consider all vessels encountered during a neck dissection as possible recipient vessel either in the current surgery or future surgery. Thus, ligation of vessels should be done as distally from origin as possible. Ligation with hemoclips is preferred by the authors because it allows for most vessel length preservation and avoids vessel twisting on itself. Ligation of vena commitans that was not utilized should also be done aiming to preserve the most length and placed such that it could be easily identified and utilized if needed.

References

1. Krol E, Brandt CT, Blakeslee-Carter J, Ahanchi SS, Dexter DJ, Karakla D, Panneton JM. Vascular interventions in head and neck cancer patients as a marker of poor survival. J Vasc Surg. 2019;69:181–9.
2. Ferlito A, Gavilan J, Buckley JG, Shaha AR, Miodonski AJ, Rinaldo A. Functional neck dissection: fact and fiction. Head Neck. 2001;23:804–8.
3. Yazici G, Sanlı TY, Cengiz M, et al. A simple strategy to decrease fatal carotid blowout syndrome after stereotactic body reirradiaton for recurrent head and neck cancers. Radiat Oncol. 2013;8:242.
4. Yamazaki H, Ogita M, Himei K, Nakamura S, Kotsuma T, Yoshida K, Yoshioka Y. Carotid blowout syndrome in pharyngeal cancer patients treated by hypofractionated stereotactic re-irradiation using CyberKnife: a multi-institutional matched-cohort analysis. Radiother Oncol. 2015;115:67–71.
5. Cengiz M, Ozyigit G, Yazici G, Dogan A, Yildiz F, Zorlu F, Gurkaynak M, Gullu IH, Hosal S, Akyol F. Salvage reirradiaton with stereotactic body radiotherapy for locally recurrent head-and-neck tumors. Int J Radiat Oncol Biol Phys. 2011;81:104–9.
6. Mccall JW, Whitaker CW, Hendershot EL. Rupture of the common carotid artery following radical neck surgery in radiated cases. AMA Arch Otolaryngol. 1959;69:431–4.

7. Dandy WE. Results following bands and ligatures on the human internal carotid artery. Ann Surg. 1946;123:384–96.
8. Elias AE, Chaudhary N, Pandey AS, Gemmete JJ. Intracranial endovascular balloon test occlusion: indications, methods, and predictive value. Neuroimaging Clin N Am. 2013;23:695–702.
9. Chang F-C, Luo C-B, Lirng J-F, Lin C-J, Lee H-J, Wu C-C, Hung S-C, Guo W-Y. Endovascular management of post-irradiated carotid blowout syndrome. PLoS One. 2015;10:e0139821.
10. Markiewicz MR, Pirgousis P, Bryant C, Cunningham JC, Dagan R, Sandhu SJ, Siragusa DA, Gopinath A, Fernandes R. Preoperative protective endovascular covered stent placement followed by surgery for management of the cervical common and internal carotid arteries with tumor encasement. J Neurol Surg B. 2017;78:052–8.
11. Wright JG, Nicholson R, Schuller DE, Smead WL. Resection of the internal carotid artery and replacement with greater saphenous vein: a safe procedure for en bloc cancer resections with carotid involvement. J Vasc Surg. 1996;23:775–82.
12. Toyoda T, Sawatari K, Yamada T, Kaneko H, Yamashita T, Taniuchi N. Endovascular therapeutic occlusion following bilateral carotid artery bypass for radiation-induced carotid artery blowout: case report. Radiat Med. 2000;18:315–7.
13. Liang NL, Guedes BD, Duvvuri U, Singh MJ, Chaer RA, Makaroun MS, Sachdev U. Outcomes of interventions for carotid blowout syndrome in patients with head and neck cancer. J Vasc Surg. 2016;63:1525–30.
14. Shumrick DA. Carotid artery rupture. Laryngoscope. 1973;83(7):1051–61.
15. Yii NW, Patel SG, Williamson P, Breach NM. Use of apron flap incision for neck dissection. Plast Reconstr Surg. 1999;103(6):1655–60. https://doi.org/10.1097/00006534-199905060-00012.
16. Heller KS, Strong EW. Carotid arterial hemorrhage after radical head and neck surgery. Am J Surg. 1979;138:607–10.
17. Maran AG, Amin M, Wilson JA. Radical neck dissection: a 19-year experience. J Laryngol Otol. 1989;103:760–4.
18. McDonald MW, Moore MG, Johnstone PAS. Risk of carotid blowout after reirradiation of the head and neck: a systematic review. Int J Radiat Oncol Biol Phys. 2012;82:1083–9.
19. Chen Y, Wang C, Wang C, Jiang R, Lin J, Liu S. Carotid blowout in patients with head and neck cancer: associated factors and treatment outcomes. Head Neck. 2015;37:265–72.
20. Genden EM, Ferlito A, Shaha AR, Talmi YP, Robbins KT, Rhys-Evans PH, Rinaldo A. Complications of neck dissection. Acta Otolaryngol. 2003;123:795–801.
21. Mirski MA, Lele AV, Fitzsimmons L, Toung TJK. Diagnosis and treatment of vascular air embolism. Anesthesiology. 2007;106:164–77.
22. Hong S, Klem C. Chapter 13: Facs hemorrhage management and vascular control. In: Textbook of military medicine: otolaryngology/head and neck surgery combat casualty care in operation Iraqi freedom and operation eduring freedom 2015. United States Government US Army; October 29, 2016:145–158.
23. Yen AJ, Conrad MB, Loftus PA, Kumar V, Nanavati SM, Wilson MW, Cooke DL. Internal jugular vein embolization to control life-threatening hemorrhage after penetrating neck trauma. J Vasc Interv Radiol. 2018;29:435–7.
24. Kondoh K, Kitahara T, Mishiro Y, Okumura S, Kubo T. Management of hemorrhagic high jugular bulb with adhesive otitis media in an only hearing ear: transcatheter endovascular embolization using detachable coils. Ann Otol Rhinol Laryngol. 2004;113:975–9.
25. Yamanaka K, Yamamoto A, Ishida K, Matsuzaki J, Ozaki T, Ishihara M, Shimahara Y, Nakajima S, Sadamitsu D, Yamasaki M. Successful endovascular therapy of a penetrating zone III jugular bulb injury. A case report. Interv Neuroradiol. 2012;18:195–9.
26. Morosanu C, Lunca S, Romedea SN, Roata C, Buga C, Ciuhodaru L. Bleeding control in stab wounds to the great vessels at the neck base. Rev Med Chir Soc Med Nat Iasi. 2005;109:559–63.
27. McCarthy CJ, Behravesh S, Naidu SG, Oklu R. Air embolism: practical tips for prevention and treatment. J Clin Med. 2016;5:93.
28. Meyer A, Gross N, Teng M. AHNS series: do you know your guidelines? Perioperative antithrombotic management in head and neck surgery. Head Neck. 2018;40:182–91.

29. Jethwa AR, Khariwala SS. When should therapeutic anticoagulation be restarted following major head and neck surgery? Laryngoscope. 2018;128:1025–6.
30. Shah-Becker S, Greenleaf EK, Boltz MM, Hollenbeak CS, Goyal N. Neck hematoma after major head and neck surgery: risk factors, costs, and resource utilization. Head Neck. 2018;40:1219–27.
31. Matory YL, Spiro RH. Wound bleeding after head and neck surgery. J Surg Oncol. 1993;53:17–9.
32. Chen Y-F, Wang T-H, Chiu Y-H, Chang D-H. Postoperative hematoma in microvascular reconstruction of the head and neck. Ann Plast Surg. 2018;80:S15–20.
33. Kucur C, Kucur C, Durmus K, et al. Management of complications and compromised free flaps following major head and neck surgery. Eur Arch Otorhinolaryngol. 2016;273:209–13.
34. Bajwa M, Tudur-Smith C, Shaw R, Schache A. Fibrin sealants in soft tissue surgery of the head and neck: a systematic review and meta-analysis of randomised controlled trials. Clin Otolaryngol. 2017;42:1141–52.
35. Huang C-W, Huang C-W, Wang C-C, et al. The impact of tissue glue in wound healing of head and neck patients undergoing neck dissection. Eur Arch Otorhinolaryngol. 2016;273:245–50.
36. Verma RK, Mathiazhagan A, Panda NK. Neck dissection with harmonic scalpel and electrocautery? A randomised study. Auris Nasus Larynx. 2016;44:590–5.
37. Borsanyi SJ. Rupture of the carotids following radical neck surgery in radiated patients. Eye Ear Nose Throat Mon. 1962;41:531–3.
38. King GD. Radical head and neck surgery in irradiated patients: complications and safeguards. Surg Clin N Am. 1965;45:567–72.
39. Cohen J, Rad I. Contemporary management of carotid blowout. Curr Opin Otolaryngol Head Neck Surg. 2004;12:110–5.
40. Powitzky R, Vasan N, Krempl G, Medina J. Carotid blowout in patients with head and neck cancer. Ann Otol Rhinol Laryngol. 2010;119:476–84.
41. Suárez C, Fernández-Alvarez V, Hamoir M, Mendenhall WM, Strojan P, Quer M, Silver CE, Rodrigo JP, Rinaldo A, Ferlito A. Carotid blowout syndrome: modern trends in management. Cancer Manag Res. 2018;10:5617–28.
42. Lu H, Chen K, Chen M, Chu P, Tai S, Wang L, Chang PM, Yang M-H. Predisposing factors, management, and prognostic evaluation of acute carotid blowout syndrome. J Vasc Surg. 2013;58:1226–35.
43. Chaloupka JC, Putman CM, Citardi MJ, Ross DA, Sasaki CT. Endovascular therapy for the carotid blowout syndrome in head and neck surgical patients: diagnostic and managerial considerations. Am J Neuroradiol. 1996;17:843.
44. Sarkar S, Mehta SA, Tiwari J, Mehta AR, Mehta MS. Complications following surgery for cancer of the larynx and pyriform fossa. J Surg Oncol. 1990;43:245–9.
45. Estomba CMC, Reinoso FAB, Velasquez AO, Macia OC, Cortés MJG, Nores JA. Carotid blowout syndrome in patients treated by larynx cancer. Braz J Otorhinolaryngol. 2017;83:653–8.
46. Jacobi C, Gahleitner C, Bier H, Knopf A. Chemoradiation and local recurrence of head and neck squamous cell carcinoma and the risk of carotid artery blowout. Head Neck. 2019;41:3073–9.
47. Timon CV, Brown D, Gullane P. Internal jugular vein blowout complicating head and neck surgery. J Laryngol Otol. 1994;108:423–5.
48. Wurster CF, Krespi YP, Sisson GA, Ossoff RH, Becker SP. A new complication of modified neck dissection: internal jugular vein blowout. Otolaryngol Head Neck Surg. 1985;93:812–4.
49. Cleland-Zamudio SS, Wax MK, Smith JD, Cohen JI. Ruptured internal jugular vein: a postoperative complication of modified/selected neck dissection. Head Neck. 2003;25:357–60.
50. Citardi MJ, Chaloupka JC, Son YH, Ariyan S, Sasaki CT. Management of carotid artery rupture by monitored endovascular therapeutic occlusion (1988-1994). Laryngoscope. 1995;105(10):1086–92. https://doi.org/10.1288/00005537-199510000-00015.
51. Bharadwaj S, Ginoya S, Tandon P, Gohel TD, Guirguis J, Vallabh H, Jevenn A, Hanouneh I. Malnutrition: laboratory markers vs nutritional assessment. Gastroenterol Rep. 2016;4:272–80.

52. Lu H-J, Chen K-W, Chen M-H, Chu P-Y, Tai S-K, Tzeng C-H, Chang PM-H, Yang M-H. Serum albumin is an important prognostic factor for carotid blowout syndrome. Jpn J Clin Oncol. 2013;43:532–9.

53. Gahleitner C, Hofauer B, Storck K, Knopf A. Outcome of carotid and subclavian blowout syndrome in patients with pharynx- and larynx carcinoma passing a standardized multidisciplinary treatment. Acta Otolaryngol. 2018;138:507–12.

54. Kerawala CJ. Complications of head and neck cancer surgery – prevention and management. Oral Oncol. 2010;46:433–5.

55. Jong MA, Candanedo C, Gross M, Cohen JE. Intervening in the acute phase of Postradiation carotid blowout syndrome. Int Arch Otorhinolaryngol. 2019;23:172–7.

56. Murros KE, Toole JF. The effect of radiation on carotid arteries: a review article. Arch Neurol. 1989;46:449–55.

57. Prasad KK, Sirsath NT, Naiknaware KV, Rani KS, Bhatia MS. Carotid blowout syndrome: an oncological emergency less discussed. South Asian J Cancer. 2017;6:85–6.

58. Chang F, Luo C, Lirng J, Lin C, Wu H, Hung S, Guo W, Teng MMH, Chang C. Evaluation of the outcomes of endovascular management for patients with head and neck cancers and associated carotid blowout syndrome of the external carotid artery. Clin Radiol. 2013;68:e561–9.

59. Huvos AG, Leaming RH, Moore OS. Clinicopathologic study of the resected carotid artery. Analysis of sixty-four cases. Am J Surg. 1973;126:570–4.

60. Ernemann U, Herrmann C, Plontke S, Schafer J, Plasswilm L, Skalej M. Pseudoaneurysm of the superior thyroid artery following radiotherapy for hypopharyngeal cancer. Ann Otol Rhinol Laryngol. 2003;112:188–90.

61. Mittal BB, Pelzer H, Tsao CS, Ward WF, Johnson P, Friedman C, Sisson GAS, Kies M. Intraoperative radiation of canine carotid artery, internal jugular vein, and vagus nerve. Therapeutic applications in the management of advanced head and neck cancers. Arch Otolaryngol Head Neck Surg. 1990;116:1425–30.

62. Cordova A, D'Arpa S, Di Lorenzo S, Toia F, Campisi G, Moschella F. Prophylactic chimera anterolateral thigh/vastus lateralis flap: preventing complications in high-risk head and neck reconstruction. J Oral Maxillofac Surg. 2014;72:1013–22.

63. Manzoor NF, Rezaee RP, Ray A, Wick CC, Blackham K, Stepnick D, Lavertu P, Zender CA. Contemporary management of carotid blowout syndrome utilizing endovascular techniques. Laryngoscope. 2017;127:383–90.

64. Osguthorpe JD, Hungerford GD. Transarterial carotid occlusion. Case report and review of literature. Arch Otolaryngol. 1984 Oct;110(10):694-6. https://doi.org/10.1001/archotol.1984.00800360066017. PMID: 6477267.

65. Razack MS, Sako K. Carotid artery hemorrhage and ligation in head and neck cancer. J Surg Oncol. 1982;19:189–92.

66. Gaba RC, West DL, Bui JT, Owens CA, Marden FA. Covered stent treatment of carotid blowout syndrome. Semin Interv Radiol. 2007;24:047–52.

67. Hanasono MM, Barnea Y, Skoracki RJ. Microvascular surgery in the previously operated and irradiated neck. Microsurgery. 2009;29:1–7.

68. Jacobson AS, Eloy JA, Park E, Roman B, Genden EM. Vessel-depleted neck: techniques for achieving microvascular reconstruction. Head Neck. 2008;30:201–7.

Neural Complications

6

Moo Hyun Kim and Antonia Kolokythas

Complications

Marginal Mandibular Nerve

In the body of oncologic literature, when evaluating nerve injuries in neck dissection, there seems to be a disproportionate amount of studies pertaining to a select few nerves, and the marginal mandibular nerve (MMN) certainly is no exception. This is to be expected, as the MMN is located at a level of the neck where neck dissections extend and perhaps is also due to its relatively superficial location.

The MMN is a branch of the cervicofacial division of cranial nerve VII with motor innervation to the muscles of facial expression. The muscles that are innervated by the marginal mandibular nerve are the orbicularis oris, depressor anguli oris, depressor labii inferioris, mentalis, and platysma muscle [1]. During neck dissection, there are various levels in the neck that may be dissected contingent on various factors such as the location of the primary tumor. The marginal mandibular branch of the facial nerve is at higher risk when removing lymph nodes in level I [2], which is divided into two separate anatomic compartments, Ia and Ib. Here, there will be a focus on level Ib, as this is where the marginal mandibular nerve is commonly encountered. The boundaries of level Ib are the mandible superiorly, anterior and posterior bellies of the digastric muscle antero-inferiorly, and the stylohyoid muscle posteriorly [3]. The anatomic contents of level Ib are wide and varied. The submandibular triangle contains the marginal mandibular, lingual nerve, and hypoglossal nerve, facial artery, and vein, perifacial lymph nodes, and submandibular gland [3].

M. H. Kim (✉) · A. Kolokythas
Department of Oral and Maxillofacial Surgery, University of Rochester – Strong Memorial Hospital, Eastman Institute for Oral Health, Rochester, NY, USA
e-mail: MooHyun_Kim@URMC.Rochester.edu;
Antonia_Kolokythas@URMC.Rochester.edu

© Springer Nature Switzerland AG 2021
T. Schlieve, W. Zaid (eds.), *Complications in Neck Dissection*,
https://doi.org/10.1007/978-3-030-62739-3_6

Particular attention must be directed to the relative location of the MMN to the fascial layer in which it is identified. The MMN is located within the superficial layer of the deep cervical fascia [4]. This nerve is located about 1 cm anterior to the angle of the mandible, and it is commonly found to cross superficial to the submandibular gland and facial vessels [5]. The submandibular gland is palpable beneath the superficial layer of the deep cervical fascia as a bulge, and when dissection leads to this gland, the fascia is incised and elevated at the inferior aspect of the gland, which is located about 2 cm below the inferior border of the mandible [3]. In a more proximal direction, once the MMN is found, it is traceable and found to turn superiorly into the parotid, where the tissue lateral and inferior to this point is safely divided to reveal the posterior belly of the digastric muscle [5].

In the setting of neck dissections, MMN injury manifests as obvious facial dysfunction. Intraoperatively, it is not sufficient to simply identify this nerve both visually and with a nerve stimulator by the operator. The astute surgeon is aware that the vitality of this nerve is quite literally in the hands of both the operator and the assistant, as overzealous manual retraction can lead to (at least) temporary nerve dysfunction [4]. Trauma to the MMN commonly results in asymmetry of the lower lip upon smiling, owing to weakness of the depressor anguli oris, depressor labii inferioris, and platysma muscle, which has secondary contributions to lip depression [2] (Fig. 6.1 MMN weakness). Interestingly, despite transection type injuries to the cervical branch of the facial nerve, with resultant platysma muscle denervation, this was found to be of little clinical importance [6].

The reported incidence of MMN injury is low. In a study by Dedivitis et al., of 708 neck dissections, 413 of which were radical and 295 that were selective, MMN injury was encountered in 39 patients, an incidence of 5.5% [7]. In another study by

Fig. 6.1 Clinical photo demonstrating effects of neuropraxia of the MMN. Weakness of the lower lip with downward turn of the corner of the mouth (right)

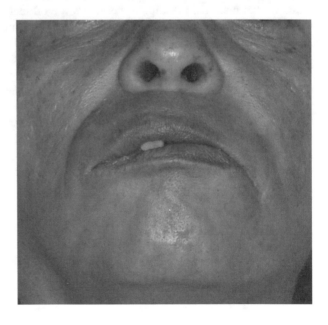

Prim et al., of 442 patients who underwent functional neck dissection, with a total of 714 neck sides operated on, the incidence of MMN injury was reported to be 1.26% [6]. Interestingly, the stage, location of the tumor, other adjunct therapies, age, and gender differences were found to influence the reported incidence rate. Patients with advanced T3 and T4 tumors, floor of mouth, nodal involvement, adjuvant radiotherapy, age under 65 years, and female gender reported a higher level of lower lip deficits [2].

In a study by Moller et al., 159 patients who underwent neck dissection with involvement of level Ib, 14% of the patients experienced MMN paresis malfunction of the lower lip 2 weeks after neck dissection. Permanent paralysis was found in 4–7% of the cases at follow-up 1–2 years later. The marked discrepancy reported between frequencies of MMN paresis at 2 weeks postoperative and at follow-up 1–2 years later is due to several factors. Axonal trauma due to likely stretching and retraction of the nerve contributes to a neurapraxia rather than outright paralysis. Recovery of the injured nerve is largely contingent on the severity of the surgical trauma. Thus, a follow-up period of at least 6 months to 1 year is advocated in order to capture the true incidence of nerve dysfunction. It is also important to note that transection of the platysma could mimic MMN paresis initially and persist until the muscle heals and function is restored [8].

Various surgical techniques are applied ranging from identification of the nerve, application of intraoperative nerve stimulation, and performing the Hayes-Martin maneuver to aid the oncologic surgeon in preserving the MMN. Identification of the nerve consists of not only direct visualization but also understanding where the nerve lies in relation to other identifiable anatomic structures, namely, the mandible and glandular structures. To prevent injury to the nerve, any incision in the neck is carried through platysma and the superficial cervical fascia and should be placed below the inferior border of the mandible at the minimum 2 cm distance [8]. Specifically, for NDs all incision designs (Aprons, Macfee, Schobinger, and their modifications) certainly meet the above criteria. Posteriorly, when the parotid tail is encountered, bluntly dissecting the parotid from the digastric muscle with superior reflection is recommended to prevent nerve injury [5]. When the submandibular gland is identified, injury to the MMN can be prevented by reflecting the superficial layer of the deep cervical fascia off the gland, with careful dissection along this plane between the facial vein and the gland [4].

Several other tools are available to help in identification and maintenance of the integrity of this structure. This requires the anesthesiologist to use non-paralytic anesthetic agents and for the surgeon to use nerve monitors and stimulators to aid in identification [6]. Another surgical method used to help avoid MMN injury is known as the Hayes-Martin maneuver, where dissection is performed anteriorly and posteriorly, facial vessels are divided and ligated, with subsequent elevation of the skin-platysma flap [5]. Of note, this technique is not always applicable in certain situations, like presence of gross disease at level Ib that requires composite resection, and thus the Hayes-Martin maneuver may not be oncologically safe, as there may be residual un-dissected lymph nodes elevated with the skin-platysma flap [9].

Management of MMN injury is largely contingent on the severity of trauma and appropriate timing. If a transection is observed intraoperatively, repair with end-to-end neurorrhaphy is recommended, but if the ends of the nerve will not come together without tension, grafting with the greater auricular or sural nerve is warranted [6]. Timing is of the utmost importance when managing nerve injuries, with conservative management in the short term (up to a certain point), to seemingly more invasive modalities as more time elapses. On follow-up, in the absence of any observed transection, if paralysis is incomplete, it is not recommended to undertake any irreversible procedures for at least 12 months, as there is a chance for spontaneous recovery [10]. In cases where there is no longer a response to electrical stimulation and integrity of the nerve is not certain, it is recommended that nerve repair be performed within 3 months, as with more time that elapses, there is an increased chance of axonal regeneration and less fibrotic degeneration [10]. Furthermore, within the 6 months of denervation, patients who are found to have muscle viability as assessed by EMG are candidates for cross facial nerve grafting (CFNG), while this same procedure is advocated in situations of denervation between 6 and 24 months only after depressor muscle viability is found to be intact via EMG [10].

After a period of 24 months, nerve grafting is no longer a viable option, and other management techniques are applied with the singular goal of achieving facial symmetry. The longer a patient is subjected to a period of denervation, there is an increased incidence of muscle fibrosis, which warrants transfer of select muscles such as the platysma and digastric muscles [10]. Of importance is to understand the limitations of this technique. After neck dissection, the platysma and digastric muscles are subject to denervation and devascularization [10]. Other management techniques that are applied are chemo-denervation of botulinum toxin to the contralateral depressor muscles, surgical myectomy, and selective marginal mandibular nerve neurectomy [10]. Again, it is important to understand the limitations of certain management considerations. Surgeons employing procedures involving neurectomy and myectomy must understand the functional and cosmetic drawbacks of these techniques, as they do require facial incisions and have the potential to leave a scar [10].

Spinal Accessory Nerve

To understand the course of the cranial nerve XI or spinal accessory in the context of neck dissections, it is important to be cognizant of the different levels in the neck where it may be encountered. Here, there will be a focus on levels II and V. The spinal accessory is found to traverse over the jugular vein, deep to the posterior belly of the digastric muscle, and then in level IIb, the nerve is found to course through lymphoid tissue [5] (Fig. 6.2 Spinal accessory nerve at level II). In level V, the spinal accessory nerve pierces the SCM and travels posteroinferiorly to innervate the trapezius muscles on its deep surface [3]. More specifically, CNXI exits the SCM deep to Erb's point and travels in level V in a relatively superficial plane to reach the anterior aspect of the trapezius muscle [5]. Anatomically, it is important to appreciate that the average distance superior to CNXI from the point where the

Fig. 6.2 CNXI prior to entering the sternocleido-mastoid muscle (CNXI displayed below)

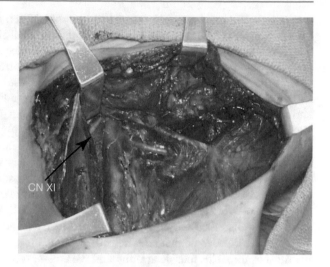

CN XI

greater auricular nerve traverses the posterior border of the SCM is ~10.7 mm. CNXI is highly vulnerable to injury after exiting the sternocleidomastoid when level V ND is performed or from overzealous retraction of the muscle [11].

An unfortunate consequence that is involved with surgical trauma to the spinal accessory nerve (SAN) is the well-documented shoulder syndrome. In this syndrome, injury to the SAN results in weakness, deformity, and pain of the shoulder girdle region and is clinically evaluated by noting weakness on shoulder shrug, limitations in abduction, flexion, and winging of the scapula at rest [12]. Despite the surgeon's best effort to protect the nerve, oftentimes there will still be resultant SAN-related deficits. There are various factors both intraoperatively and postoperatively that contribute to this dreaded sequela. During neck dissections, overzealous retraction, compression, thermal energy emitted by electrocautery, and inadvertent ligation of the SAN are contributing factors to SAN injury, while in the postoperative period, bleeding, hematoma formation, infections, and scars can result in axonotmesis and neurapraxia type injuries [13]. To further highlight the issue of resultant SAN damage despite the surgeon's deliberate attempts at sparing the SAN is the concept of devascularization. In level IIb dissection, the lymphatic tissue is mobilized and passed under the nerve. During this time, overzealous skeletonization of CNXI will result in devascularization and subsequent axonal injury, leading to shoulder syndrome [14].

There exists a cascade or domino like effect that is inherent with SAN injuries primarily due to the delicate interplay between different nerves and the mechanics of adjacent muscles and bones. From an innervation standpoint, it is important to note that the trapezius muscle is not solely innervated by CNXI. In a study by Karaman et al., it was found that the cervical plexus provides the following levels of contribution to the trapezius muscle: large contribution in 10%, moderate in 43%, and a very small contribution in 47% of patients [13]. However, in a study by Mcgarvey et al., it was pointed out that the contribution of the cervical plexus to the trapezius is still much less compared with that of CNXI motor supply [15]. From a biomechanical standpoint, it is vital to note the mechanistic relations between different structures that, in aggregate, contribute to shoulder syndrome. To further the domino like metaphor, after neck dissection, when the trapezius muscle is denervated to varying degrees, weakness ensues, which causes the scapula to drop and take on a winged formation, which in turn causes reduced glenohumeral abduction and flexion, and ultimately results in decreased shoulder function, increased pain, and decreased overall quality of life [16].

When evaluating the recovery potential after CNXI injury, the most prognostic indicator is the degree of injury inflicted. From most severe axonal injury to least, neurotmesis was found to have the worst outcome, while axonotmesis was described to have recovery periods extending to 18 months, and neurapraxia with the most expedient recovery, taking an average of 6–8 weeks [15]. When the SAN has been stretched or disturbed but is largely intact, effectively an axonotmesis type nerve injury, it was discovered that after neck dissection, immediate signs of nerve injury, manifest as trapezius muscle atrophy and weakness, were not apparent and did not present until weeks later, as there is thought to be axoplasmic flow that may persist distal to the nerve injury, which aids in muscle tone [15]. This discovery has useful clinical implications, as many patients after neck dissection are not likely to manifest any shoulder movement deficits prior to discharge and supports the notion that postoperative physiotherapy following axonotmesis will take at minimum 3 months to observe any effects [15].

Upon initial evaluation of the literature regarding SAN injury, the reported incidence is rather high. In a study by Mcgarvey et al., even when the nerve is deliberately spared, SAN injury occurred in 67% of patients but with gradual improvement in shoulder dysfunction and pain reported over a 12-month period [16]. Shoulder syndrome was reported in 30% of patients who underwent functional neck dissection, in 50% of patients who underwent modified neck dissection, and in 60% of patients who underwent radical neck dissection [17]. Furthermore, in the study by Dedivitis et al., when conducting a survey of 65 patients who underwent neck dissection and a follow-up period of 1.6 years, 23% did not report any shoulder dysfunction, 54% endorsed mild shoulder dysfunction, 15% reported moderate shoulder dysfunction, and 8% stated that they suffered severe shoulder dysfunction [7]. These results amount to a staggering 77% of patients reporting some level of shoulder dysfunction.

In another study by Wilgen et al., it was found that "dysfunction of the spinal accessory nerve occurs in all cases after neck dissection with resection of the nerve and in about 22% when it is preserved" and shoulder "pain may also be present in 49% of the cases without signs of dysfunction" [18]. It should be noted however, that shoulder syndrome does not occur in all patients even when the SAN is sacrificed, and as such, preservation of the nerve does not necessarily indicate that the patient will not have any deficits in the postoperative period [4].

Despite the high rates of neural complications reported above, there are other studies that reveal just the opposite. In a study by Prim et al., paralysis of the 11th nerve occurred in 12 cases (1.68%) [6]. And in another study by Dedivitis et al., injury to the accessory nerve was observed in 5.1% of the radical neck dissections performed [7]. There are various reasons to explain the seemingly conflicting reported incidences of injury to the SAN. As an example, when electromyography is used to determine the extent of nerve damage, there is a higher percentage of spinal accessory nerve dysfunction reported [6]. Surgical technique and instrumentation were also influential in impacting the level of shoulder dysfunction experienced in the postoperative period. There was enhanced recovery of shoulder function with use of the harmonic scalpel versus electrocautery, as electrocautery creates more thermal dissipation, and subsequent injury to the SAN [19].

The various techniques described in the oncologic literature to aid in preventing damage to the spinal accessory centers not only around successful identification of the nerve but also the ability to understand the relative geographic topography in the area of interest. CNXI is found to enter the sternocleidomastoid muscle about two finger breadths inferior to the posterior belly of the digastric muscle, and its identification is further aided by electrocautery (when the patient is not paralyzed), as the nerve is stimulated, shoulder jumping will be present [5]. Another anatomic landmark to be cognizant of is the internal jugular vein in the anterior triangle, as this is an area where the SAN traverses the "vein ventrally in 56% of cases and dorsally in 44%" [11]. After successful identification of the nerve, it is important to "not injure the SAN during elevation of the skin flaps posteriorly since the nerve exits the posterior aspect of the SCM in a subcutaneous plane" and the nerve is further isolated by "blunt spreading of tissue in the direction of the nerve's course, and it is dissected from its entry point to the SCM cephalad to the level of the posterior belly of the digastric muscle" [4]. At the level of the trapezius muscle, care must be taken to not mistake the levator scapulae as the trapezius during elevation of the flap, as this "mistake may lead to inadvertent transection of not only the eleventh nerve but also the nerves to the levator scapulae, resulting in shoulder disability" [5].

Management of patients with SAN injury begins with a thorough examination after neck dissection. The clinical examination after neck dissection should specifically include assessment for shoulder drop, muscle atrophy, and active abduction [18]. Despite this unfavorable outlook in situations where neurotmesis has occurred, intraoperative repair is typically undertaken. When managing situations in the setting of spinal accessory nerve transection, two management techniques are primary anastomosis of the transected nerve endings and preservation of the branches of C2, C3, and C4, as doing so has shown to help in improvement with shoulder range of motion, and postoperatively should shoulder dysfunction manifest. Physical therapy is an adjunct tool to help with reducing pain and to help improve the patient's quality of life [6]. In addition to the measures described above taken to help with nerve recovery, there exists therapies to help with not just recovery but regeneration at the molecular level. In a study by Barber et al., brief electrical stimulation (BES) was used to improve neuronal regeneration modulation of brain-derived neurotrophic growth factor (BDNF) pathways. BES was mostly effective in improvement of shoulder dysfunction for patients undergoing ND that included levels IIb and V [14].

Lingual Nerve/Hypoglossal Nerves

Injury to the lingual nerve can occur when the parasympathetic fibers from the lingual nerve to the submandibular ganglion are transected, which is an essential step for mobilization of the submandibular gland during dissection at level Ib. Wide retraction of the posterior border of the mylohyoid muscle and visualization of the nerve, which is usually tented down as a "V" by its attachment to the gland, is crucial during this maneuver to avoid transection of the lingual nerve. The hypoglossal nerve runs deep to the belly of the digastric and deep to the hyoglossus muscle, so it is usually not at risk (Fig. 6.3). However, it is often accompanied by small veins that bleed easily. Careless use of the bovie at the posterior-inferior border of the gland can damage the nerve. In any case of witnessed nerve transection, immediate repair should be undertaken. Alternatively, use of interpositional graft and nerve protectors to promote nerve regeneration are crucial steps in recovery.

Great Auricular Nerve

The great auricular nerve is unique among the various other nerves encountered in neck dissections due to its relatively superficial location. The nerve originating from the cervical plexus, at the levels of C2 and C3, is responsible for providing sensation to the skin overlying the lower aspect of the pinna and angle of the mandible [20]. More specifically, the great auricular nerve is found to course obliquely over the sternocleidomastoid muscle, parallel and slightly posterior to the external jugular vein [5].

The sequela of great auricular nerve injury is numbness. Because the great auricular nerve innervates the auricle, damage to the nerve results in hypoesthesia, which can be an issue for patients [5]. Despite decreased sensation to the auricle as being

Fig. 6.3 Hypoglossal nerve running deep to the posterior belly of the digastric muscle

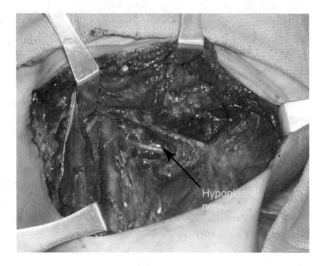

a commonly reported consequence of nerve damage, pain is another symptom that is characterized. Formation of a neuroma can create a trigger point on the neck and result in migraine-type pain symptoms on the face [21]. In the setting of neck dissections, there is a dearth of data on great auricular nerve injury. But, in the context of rhytidectomies, great auricular nerve injury is reported to be as high as 6–7% [22].

The literature is quite robust regarding specific anatomical metrics employed when attempting to avoid injury to the great auricular nerve (GAN). In Lefkowitz et al., it was discovered that the "GAN at its most superficial location was found to be consistently at a ratio of one-third the distance from either the mastoid process or the external auditory canal to the clavicular origin of the SCM" [22]. Another metric for point of reference is described in a study by Murphy et al., in which the "posterior borders of the platysma and EJV are found, on average, 0.08 cm away from each other, and the free edge of the platysma was most often posterior to the EJV" and "the distance from the platysma to the GAN was, on average, 0.60 cm" and "the distance between the EJV and the GAN was 1.17 cm" [20]. Awareness of specific measurements is certainly useful during surgery but does not seem entirely pragmatic at times [3]. Injury to the great auricular nerve can be managed by surgical exploration attempt to nerve release and provide decompression [21].

Cervical Plexus

The cervical plexus is derived from spinal nerves C1 through C4 and is responsible for sensation on the skin of the neck, the ear, and behind the ear [1]. Injury to the cervical plexus results not only in sensory deficits, namely to the regions of the ear and neck, but contributes to a well-documented syndrome that was discussed above in the section encompassing the spinal accessory nerve. Damage to the cervical plexus contributes to the pathogenesis of the shoulder syndrome that includes lesions of the cervical motor branches for the trapezius muscle (C2-C4), the levator scapulae (C3-C5), and the supraclavicular nerves (C3-C4) [17]. Primary consideration of preservation of the cervical plexus during neck dissection involves identification of the plexus and fascial sparing. Once the cervical plexus is found, it is recommended to avoid dissecting the cervical plexus off the deep muscles and, furthermore, aim for preservation of the cervical rootlets where they exit between the middle and the anterior scalene muscles [3, 5].

Brachial Plexus

When studying the anatomy of the brachial plexus, it is imperative to understand the various subdivisions of the nerve. The brachial plexus is derived from the ventral rami of C5-T1 spinal nerves and consists of roots, trunks, and cords that lie deep to a dense layer of prevertebral fascia [23]. These subdivisions are further grouped into a supraclavicular and infraclavicular branches, where supraclavicular branches arise from the roots or trunks, and infraclavicular branches arise from the cords

[23]. Damage to the brachial plexus has effects on arm strength along with sensory alterations. Injury to C5 and C6 results in both sensory deficits over the lateral portion of the upper arm and weakness of the biceps, brachial, and deltoid muscles, which may result in an Erb-Duchenne deformity, characterized by left arm extension and pronation of the forearm [23]. Prevention and careful dissection around the rootlets are the best ways to avoid injuries.

Phrenic Nerve

Understanding the relative anatomy of the phrenic nerve requires knowledge of its origins and the levels of the neck where the phrenic nerve is encountered. The phrenic nerve is derived from the ventral primary rami of C3-C5 (cervical plexus) and gives off pericardial branches and innervates the diaphragm [1]. The nerve is encountered in levels IV and V during neck dissection and crosses over the anterior scalene muscle immediately anterior to the brachial plexus and lies immediately under the enveloping fascia of the anterior scalene muscles [5].

Phrenic nerve injury may result in a compromised respiratory status. The degree of nerve injury directly correlates to the degree of pulmonary compromise. In cases of neurapraxia, there may be temporary diaphragmatic paralysis, whereas in neurotmesis, permanent diaphragmatic paralysis may result [24]. In many instances, nerve injury is uncommon enough, that it oftentimes is not noticed, and an alternative method to even know there was trauma to the nerve is to obtain a chest X-ray, which may show lung infiltrates and atelectasis [7]. Furthermore, postoperative imaging may reveal elevation of the affected hemi-diaphragm with decreased lung volumes [3].

There is a lack of data within the literature regarding the incidence of phrenic nerve injury after neck dissection. It may be postulated that the reason for this lack of reported damage may be due to the dissection that is typically superficial to the deep cervical and prevertebral fascia thus affording avoidance of injury to the nerve [4].

There are different management recommendations based on severity of the initial injury. In cases where there is transient paralysis of the diaphragm, observation is recommended as there may be spontaneous recovery that occurs anywhere from 3 days to 6 months [24]. In situations where there is bilateral phrenic paralysis, this is deemed a serious complication and may lead to respiratory failure and the need for mechanical ventilation [1].

Vagus Nerve

Within the carotid sheath, the vagus nerve is in close approximation to both the carotid artery and internal jugular vein running in a grove between the great vessels [5] (Fig. 6.4). Injury to the vagus nerve during neck dissection results in voice changes, and in dire circumstances, aspiration. Within the setting of radical neck

Fig. 6.4 Vagus nerve
within the carotid sheath

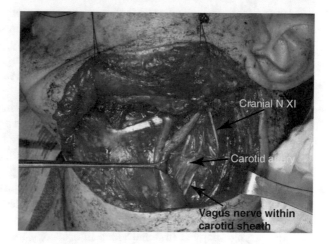

dissections, when the internal jugular vein is ligated, the vagus nerve is prone to injury, and if the injury occurs below the nodose ganglion, it results in vocal fold paralysis and if the injury occurs above, there is also dysphagia and aspiration [7]. The reported incidence of damage to the vagus nerve within the context of radical neck dissections is described as a complication that can and should be avoided as the nerve can usually be visualized between the great vessels and protected (Fig. 6.4) [1]. When performing radical neck dissections, the internal jugular vein is dissected in its entirety prior to ligation, as the vagus is especially prone to damage during ligation of this vessel [4]. Further techniques that can be employed to decrease risk of damage to the vagus nerve is to identify the nerve, protect it, avoid unnecessary manipulation of the carotid sheath, and judicious application of any electrocautery near the nerve [25].

As with many postoperative management protocols instituted in medicine, the most conservative options are exhausted first before advancing to more invasive choices, and the management of vagus nerve injuries is no exception. If a transection is observed intraoperatively, initial nerve repair should be attempted, but if the injury was a crush injury, observation and treatment of complications are recommended [25]. As discussed above, vagus nerve injuries present with unique challenges that include voice changes, dysphagia, and aspiration.

Superior Laryngeal Nerve

When performing dissections in the vicinity of the carotid vessels, careful attention must be paid to the proximity of the superior laryngeal nerve. This nerve stems from the vagus nerve and travels inferior and medial to the upper portion of the larynx and passes posterior to the internal and external carotid arteries [25].

The sequela of damage to the superior laryngeal nerve ranges from voice changes to aspiration. When the superior laryngeal nerve is injured, there is paralysis of the cricothyroid muscle, with resultant changes in phonation at a high pitch, and bilateral damage to the internal branch of the nerve results in sensory loss to the laryngeal membrane, with catastrophic consequences, namely, aspiration [25].

The reported incidence of injury to the superior laryngeal nerve is varied. There are reported rates of temporary paralysis lower than 5.1% and permanent paralysis around 2% [26].

A particularly useful anatomic landmark to help aid in preventing injury to this nerve is the superior thyroid artery. The superior thyroid artery is the first branch of the external carotid system and loops slightly superiorly before beginning its inferior transit toward the superior pole of the thyroid gland, and it is precisely at this level that "it is close to the superior laryngeal nerve" [5].

The first step to successful management of nerve injuries is a thorough postoperative clinical examination. In patients who are suspected of having sustained such vagal injuries, screening for dysphagia, a breathy voice, and frequent cough should undergo laryngoscopy at first and video fluoroscopy for a more complete detailed examination to document vocal cord paralysis (adductor), cricopharyngeal dysfunction, or both [25].

Cervical Sympathetic Chain

The cervical sympathetic chain is located close to the carotid vessels. More specifically, the chain is located deep, posterior, and medial to the carotid artery and found between the prevertebral fascia and the carotid sheath [6]. Cervical sympathetic chain contributes innervation to various structures that include vascular smooth muscles, erector pili, sweat glands of upper neck and face, vascular smooth muscles of orbit, forehead, upper nasal cavity, and dilator pupillae [1].

The adverse consequence of damage to the cervical sympathetic chain has implications from both a functional and cardiac standpoint. Damage to this sympathetic chain results in a well-known phenomenon, namely, Bernard-Horner syndrome or oculosympathetic paresis characterized by ptosis, miosis, and anhidrosis [7]. The cardiac effects from damage to the sympathetic fibers are presented as prolonged Q-T interval with resulting tachyarrhythmias [1].

The incidence of damage to these sympathetic fibers is rather low. In a study by Dedivitis et al., damage to the cervical sympathetic chain was found to have occurred in three sides in our series [7]. As is the case with neck dissections, the best technique is early identification and avoidance. Horner's syndrome is often a result of manipulation and traction "in or around the carotid sheath" [6]. The management for Horner's syndrome is conservative. Intraoperatively, when the cervical sympathetic chain is identified, care must be taken to avoid heavy traction and stretching, while postoperatively, if Horner's syndrome manifests, supportive ophthalmic care is required along with appropriate follow-up [6].

In conclusion, neurological injuries during neck dissection are preventable with adherence to good surgical techniques. In-depth knowledge and understanding of the special anatomy coupled with experience will allow the surgeon to avoid damage to CNs that can be devastating to the patients' quality of life.

References

1. Talmi YP. Minimizing complications in neck dissection. J Laryngol Otol. 1999;113(2):101–13.
2. Batstone MD, Scott B, Lowe D, Rogers SN. Marginal mandibular nerve injury during neck dissection and its impact on patient perception of appearance. Head Neck. 2009;31(5):673–8.
3. Morlandt ABHJ. Surgical management of the neck. In: Atlas of operative oral and maxillofacial surgery. John Wiley & Sons, Inc. editorial offices in Ames, Iowa; West Sussex, UK; Oxford, UK. 2015. p. 424–30.
4. Bagheri SC, Bell RB, Khan HA, Duncan L, Dolan J, Sprehe C, et al. Current therapy in oral and maxillofacial surgery. St. Louis: Elsevier Saunders; 2012.
5. Eibling DE. Neck dissections. In: Operative otolaryngology: head and neck surgery, vol. 1; Saunders United States. 1997. p. 676–718.
6. Prim MP, De Diego JI, Verdaguer JM, Sastre N, Rabanal I. Neurological complications following functional neck dissection. Eur Arch Otorhinolaryngol. 2006;263(5):473–6.
7. Dedivitis RA, Guimaraes AV, Pfuetzenreiter EG, Jr., Castro MA. [Neck dissection complications]. Braz J Otorhinolaryngol. 2011;77(1):65–9.
8. Moller MN, Sorensen CH. Risk of marginal mandibular nerve injury in neck dissection. Eur Arch Otorhinolaryngol. 2012;269(2):601–5.
9. Tirelli G, Bergamini PR, Scardoni A, Gatto A, Boscolo Nata F, Marcuzzo AV. Intraoperative monitoring of marginal mandibular nerve during neck dissection. Head Neck. 2018;40(5):1016–23.
10. Murthy SP, Paderno A, Balasubramanian D. Management of the marginal mandibular nerve during and after neck dissection. Curr Opin Otolaryngol Head Neck Surg. 2019;27(2):104–9.
11. Bater MC, Dufty J, Brennan PA. High division of the accessory nerve: a rare anatomical variation as a possible pitfall during neck dissection surgery. J Cranio-Maxillofac Surg. 2005;33(5):340–1.
12. Witt RL, Rejto L. Spinal accessory nerve monitoring in selective and modified neck dissection. Laryngoscope. 2007;117(5):776–80.
13. Karaman M, Tek A, Cl U, Akduman D, Bi laç Ö. Effect of functional neck dissection and post-operative radiotherapy on the spinal accessory nerve. Acta Otolaryngol. 2009;129(8):872–80.
14. Barber B, Seikaly H, Ming Chan K, Beaudry R, Rychlik S, Olson J, et al. Intraoperative brief electrical stimulation of the spinal accessory nerve (BEST SPIN) for prevention of shoulder dysfunction after oncologic neck dissection: a double-blinded, randomized controlled trial. J Otolaryngol Head Neck Surg. 2018;47(1):7–10.
15. McGarvey AC, Chiarelli PE, Osmotherly PG, Hoffman GR, Eisele DW. Physiotherapy for accessory nerve shoulder dysfunction following neck dissection surgery: a literature review. Head Neck. 2011;33(2):274–80.
16. McGarvey AC, Hoffman GR, Osmotherly PG, Chiarelli PE. Maximizing shoulder function after accessory nerve injury and neck dissection surgery: a multicenter randomized controlled trial. Head Neck. 2015;37(7):1022–31.
17. Salerno G, Cavaliere M, Foglia A, Pellicoro DP, Mottola G, Nardone M, et al. The 11th nerve syndrome in functional neck dissection. Laryngoscope. 2002;112(7):1299–307.
18. van Wilgen CP, Dijkstra PU, van der Laan BFAM, Plukker JT, Roodenburg JLN. Shoulder complaints after neck dissection; is the spinal accessory nerve involved? Br J Oral Maxillofac Surg. 2003;41(1):7–11.
19. Mathialagan AMS, Verma RKMSDNBM, Panda NKMSFF. Comparison of spinal accessory dysfunction following neck dissection with harmonic scalpel and electrocautery – a randomized study. Oral Oncol. 2016;61:142–5.
20. Murphy R, Dziegielewski P, O'Connell D, Seikaly H, Ansari K. The great auricular nerve: an anatomic and surgical study. J Otolaryngol Head Neck Surg. 2012;41(1):S75–S7.
21. Barbour JR, Gontre G, Halpern D. Surgical decompression of the greater auricular nerve: a therapeutic option in neurapraxia following rhytidectomy. Plast Reconstr Surg. 2012;130:41.

22. Lefkowitz T, Hazani R, Chowdhry S, Elston J, Yaremchuk MJ, Wilhelmi BJ. Anatomical landmarks to avoid injury to the great auricular nerve during rhytidectomy. Aesthet Surg J. 2013;33(1):19–23.
23. Monteiro MJ, Altman K, Khandwala A. Injury to the brachial plexus in neck dissections. Br J Oral Maxillofac Surg. 2009;48(3):197–8.
24. Yaddanapudi S, Shah SC. Bilateral phrenic nerve injury after neck dissection: an uncommon cause of respiratory failure. J Laryngol Otol. 1996;110(3):281–3.
25. AbuRahma AF, Lim RY. Management of vagus nerve injury after carotid endarterectomy. Surgery. 1996;119(3):245–7.
26. Giulea C, Enciu O, Toma EA, Martin S, Fica S, Miron A. Total thyroidectomy for malignancy – is central neck dissection a risk factor for recurrent nerve injury and postoperative hypocalcemia? A tertiary center experience in Romania. Acta Endocrinol. 2019;15(1):80–5.

Complications Related to Radical Neck Dissections and Management of Recurrent Neck Disease

7

Fawaz Alotaibi, Ricardo Lugo, D. David Kim, and Ghali E. Ghali

Introduction

With the exclusion of distant metastases, the most important prognostic factor in the treatment of patients with squamous cell carcinoma (SCCa) of the head and neck is the status of cervical lymph nodes [1, 2, 4, 7]. The presence of one single lymph node, with metastatic cancer, reduces survival by 50%, and contralateral or bilateral nodal involvement reduces survival by an additional 50% [1, 8]. Therefore, appropriate management of cervical node metastasis is critical in the overall planning and treatment of squamous cell carcinoma of the upper aerodigestive tract [4]. In this chapter, we will discuss the history and the development of the radical neck dissection (RND) and modified radical neck dissection (MRND), indications, classifications, and complications and review the management of recurrent neck disease.

In the nineteenth century, surgeons realized that the spread of head and neck cancer to the cervical lymph nodes signified a poor prognosis [1, 4]. In January 1888, Franciszek Jawdyn'ski, a Polish surgeon, performed a radical en bloc neck dissection, a surgical procedure that remained globally unknown despite being published in a Polish journal – the *Gazeta Lekarska* [3, 4, 9, 10]. That patient was then presented six weeks later at the meeting of the Medical Society of Warsaw [3, 4, 9, 11].

F. Alotaibi (✉) · R. Lugo · D. D. Kim
Department of Oral and Maxillofacial Surgery, Head and Neck Oncology/Microvascular Reconstruction, Louisiana State University Health Sciences Center at Shreveport, Shreveport, LA, USA
e-mail: falota@lsuhsc.edu; rlugo@lsuhsc.edu; DKim1@lsuhsc.edu

G. E. Ghali
Department of Oral and Maxillofacial Surgery, Head and Neck Oncology, Louisiana State University Health Sciences Center at Shreveport, Shreveport, LA, USA
e-mail: GGhali@lsuhsc.edu

© Springer Nature Switzerland AG 2021
T. Schlieve, W. Zaid (eds.), *Complications in Neck Dissection*,
https://doi.org/10.1007/978-3-030-62739-3_7

111

George Washington Crile was the first surgeon who systematically described the technique of radical neck dissection in one paper in 1905 and in another paper in 1906 [12, 13]. The latter article is still considered to be one of the landmark articles in the head and neck literature [5, 12, 13]. With his description of 132 cases, he advocated the removal of the lymph nodes in the neck along with the sternocleido-mastoid muscle (SCM), internal jugular vein (IJV), and spinal accessory nerve (SAN). He established the technique of radical neck dissection (RND) [5, 13]. Notwithstanding, in his article, he reported that if the accessory nerve is not directly involved by cancer, it might be preserved. He thought about the morbidity of the RND and provided a guide to the modified radical neck dissection (MRND) [1–5, 13].

Dr. Hayes Martin from Memorial Hospital in New York neck dissection mim-icked the original radical neck dissection but extended to include omohyoid muscle, submandibular gland, the tail of the parotid gland, and most of the cervical plexus nerves [1–3, 14]. In an article published in *Cancer* in 1951, in which he analyzed 1450 cases, Dr. Martin emphasized that "any technique that is designed to preserve the spinal accessory nerve should be condemned unequivocally" and "routine pro-phylactic neck dissection is considered illogical and unacceptable" for cancer of the oral cavity with the exception if a transcervical approach was required [3, 14]. His other indications for radical neck dissection included, definite clinical evidence that cancer is present in the cervical lymphatics, primary control of lesion giving rise to the neck metastasis in a separate procedure or with the RND while having a reason-able chance of complete removal of the neck disease and having no clinical or roent-genographic evidence of distant metastasis, his final indication for the RND is that this procedure should offer a superior chance of cure when compared radiation therapy [14].

Despite the RND success in neck disease control, many surgeons were concerned about the significant long-term morbidity associated with this procedure, including shoulder dysfunction, cosmetic deformity, cutaneous paraesthesia, chronic neck, and shoulder pain syndrome, and massive facial edema with bilateral RNDs [1–3]. The first original systematic approach to functional neck dissection (FND) was pub-lished by Osvaldo Sua'rez, an Argentinean surgeon, in 1963 [15]. Sua'rez is genu-inely the 'father' of functional neck dissection [2]. He described that cervical lymphatics are contained within fascial compartments that can be removed while preserving important structures and minimizing the morbidity of RND and obtain-ing regional control [1, 2, 15]. Sua'rez technique of FND gained popularity and was adopted by many surgeons like Bocca and Ce'sar Gavila'n and was recognized as an effective technique to the English literature [1, 3, 16–24].

With a better understanding of the lymphatic drainage system in the head and neck, in 1960, Ballantyne, MD Anderson, popularized the concept of MRND and selective neck dissection (SND). Only the lymph node groups with the highest risk of metastasis based on the location of the primary tumor were removed [3, 25].

The RND remains the primary reference procedure for neck dissection, with all other neck dissections representing one or more modifications of this procedure

(Fig. 7.1). The RND boundaries include superiorly the inferior border of the mandible and the skull base; inferiorly the clavicle; medially the sternohyoid muscle, hyoid bone, and contralateral anterior belly of the digastric muscle; and laterally the anterior border of the trapezius muscle. The dissection includes levels I through V, SCM, IJV, SAN, and submandibular salivary gland [1]. The indications for RND are summarized in Table 7.1 [5].

In general, there are no major contraindications for RND; however, tumors that invade the skull base or those with massive extension of the disease into the parapharyngeal space, prevertebral musculature, or extension of the disease into the deep lobe of the parotid gland may be tagged as "inoperable tumors," a term that has been replaced with "very advanced disease." Neck disease involving the common carotid artery remains controversial; generally, the sacrifice of the carotid artery along with neck dissection is potentially an uncurable situation due to the disease not limited only to the carotid artery but also involving surrounding structures such as the vagus nerve, scalene muscles, and parapharyngeal musculature. Sacrifice of

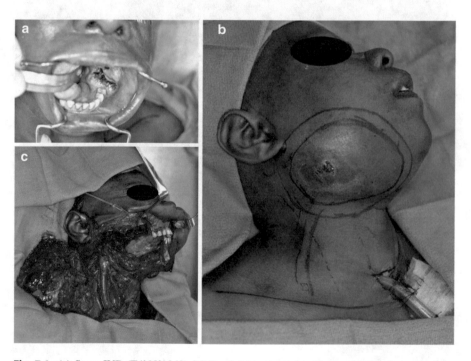

Fig. 7.1 (a) Stage IVB (T4bN3bM0) SCCa of right retromolar trigone. (b) Involvement of the facial skin and design of the planned resection with radical neck dissection. (c) Composite resection including right segmental mandibulectomy with disarticulation, right posterior maxillectomy, right pharyngectomy, and right radical neck dissection. (d) Right modified neck dissection including levels I-V, spinal accessory nerve, sternocleidomastoid muscle, and internal jugular vein. (e) Fibular free flap to reconstruct the mandible and the intraoral soft tissue defect. (f) Anterolateral thigh (ALT) free flap to reconstruct the facial defect. Note: the advancement in microvascular reconstruction allowed for more aggressive radical resection

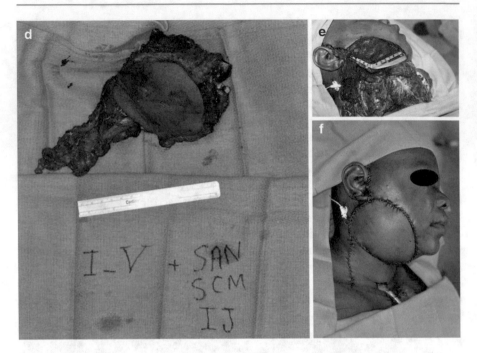

Fig. 7.1 (continued)

Table 7.1 Indication for RND and MRND

N3 neck disease, especially in the upper neck
Bulky metastatic disease near the accessory nerve
Tumor directly involving the accessory nerve
Multiple clinically palpable nodes, especially near the accessory nerve (N2b, N2c)
Recurrent metastatic tumor after previous radiation therapy
Recurrent disease in the neck after previous neck dissection
Salvage surgery in patients with previous chemoradiation therapy, especially in those who presented with bulky or level II nodal disease
Involvement of the platysma or skin, requiring a sacrifice of a portion of skin in the upper neck
Clinical signs of apparent extranodal disease

the common carotid artery and appropriate reconstruction may be technically possible; however, the recurrence rate is still extremely high, with average survival rates in these patients measured in months [5].

The MRND involves the preservation of one or more non-lymphatic structures routinely sacrificed in an RND. The standard is to name preserved structures in the description of the operation (e.g., MRND with preservation of SAN) [1]. Some authors subdivide MRND into type I (preservation of the SAN), type II (preservation of SAN and SCM), and type III (preservation of SCM, SAN, and IJV) [6]. The indications for MRND are the same as RND [1]; however, the decision to preserve or sacrifice any specific structure must be justified. The most performed MRND for SCCa with palpable neck metastasis is MRND preserving the SAN (type I) [1] [Fig. 7.2].

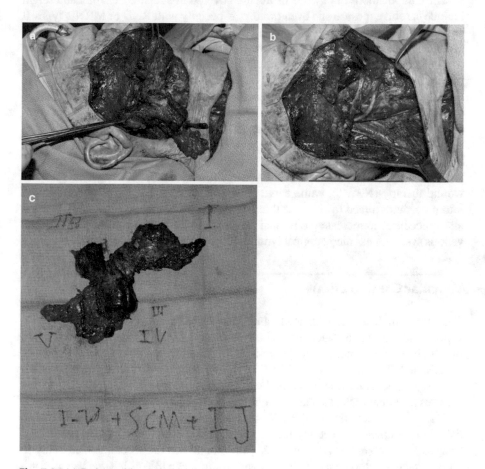

Fig. 7.2 (a) Patient with recurrent neck disease s/p CXRT for unknown primary (rcTxN1M0). Patient underwent modified radical neck dissection (MRND) with preservation of spinal accessory nerve. (b) Modified radical neck dissection (MRND) with preservation of spinal accessory nerve utilizing MacFee incision. (c) Modified radical neck dissection (MRND) levels I-V, sternocleido-mastoid muscle, and internal jugular vein

Chyle Complications

Chylous fistula is a well-recognized but uncommon complication of RND and MRND [26, 27, 30]. The literature reports the rates of these complications ranging from 0.62% to 6.2% with a higher incidence associated with the bilateral neck dissection [28, 29, 31]. It is well established that chyle complications are more common on the left side than the right side [28, 32].

The complications of chylous fistula are covered in a separate chapter and might include carotid exposure and even rupture, especially with RND or MRND types II and III. The delay in the healing process may subsequently lead to the formation of orocutaneous or pharyngocutaneous fistulae. Moreover, this complication may lead to a delay in postoperative adjuvant therapy and affect overall survival. Other complication includes the formation of chylothorax when the chylous fluid collects in the pleural cavity [27]. The consequences of these complications can be mild to severe and even life threatening. Therefore, prevention is the key, and prompt identification and management are necessary [28].

In general, conservative management of chylous and thoracic duct injuries following neck dissections is the first line of treatment. Nonsurgical treatment includes nutritional approaches, somatostatin analogs (octreotide), and negative pressure wound therapy (NPWT), while surgical management can be broadly categorized into procedures aimed to close the thoracic duct such as thoracic duct embolization and procedures to recreate the normal physiologic flow from the lymphatic to the venous system, i.e., microsurgical lymphatic–venous anastomoses [28].

Vascular Complications

Vascular complications with RND and MRND can be broadly categorized into venous and arterial complications. The venous complications are mainly related to the sacrifice of the internal jugular vein (IJV) during bilateral RND. Anomalies of the IJV, including duplications of the IJV where it bifurcate to two separate branches with separate connection proximally and fenestrations, where bifurcation that reunites proximal to the subclavian vein has been reported [33–37].

The bilateral sacrifice of the IJVs and its potential complications were established in the nineteenth century [38]. Leclerc and Roy were the first to recommend "staged ligation" of the IJVs in 1932. One month was the recommended delay to allow for the development of collateral venous drainage [38–40]. Razack et al. compared the complications of single-staged and two-staged approaches and found that two-stage complications occurred at rates of 3–30% as opposed to 5–63% in single-staged approaches [38, 49]. However, Ahn and Sindelar reported no statistical significance in the reduction in morbidity and mortality between the staged or simultaneous sacrifice of bilateral IJVs [41].

The bilateral sacrifice of IJVs can significantly compromise the cerebral outflow, by increasing the intracranial pressure (ICP) [38, 42–44] resulting in physiological changes like systemic hypertension, facial edema 54%, laryngeal edema with respiratory distress, syndrome of inappropriate antidiuretic hormone secretion (SIADH), ophthalmoplegia, blindness, and stroke [38, 45–51]. The IJVs are the predominant cerebral outflow tracts, with 80% of the population having a right-sided dominant IJV [38, 43, 51, 52]. Moreover, usually following sacrifice of bilateral IJVs, the predominant outflow is mediated through the external vertebral plexus [38, 53]. Other outflow tracts include pterygoid plexus and orbital plexus [38, 51, 52]. As a general rule, whenever possible, bilateral radical neck dissections should be done with preservation of one internal jugular vein [41].

Several reports discussed the immediate reconstruction of at least one of the IJVs following bilateral radical neck dissection to minimize postoperative complications [54, 55]. Katsuno et al. reported three types of IJV reconstruction – type A: *internal jugular vein–external jugular vein anastomosis; type B: bypass grafting (internal jugular vein–internal jugular vein); and type C: bypass grafting (internal jugular vein–external jugular vein)* [55]. Kamizono et al. reported another modification and called it type K, in which the anastomosis between the internal jugular vein and the anterior jugular vein was performed without disturbing the external jugular vein as to maintain the facial outflow and subsequently minimize the postoperative facial edema [54].

Some investigators evaluated the patency of the preserved IJV. Fisher et al. reported several risk factors for thrombosis of the IJV: (1) the vessel may be damaged during the dissection, (2) devascularization of the vessel wall may increase the risk of transmural injury, (3) ligation of the branches might produce blind pouches or ligation too close to the IVJ, which may narrow the vessel, and (4) the surface of the vein may become desiccated [56]. They concluded that FND is a safe procedure when performed bilaterally or with contralateral RND in a single-stage operation with the resection of the primary tumor [56]. Makiguch et al. evaluated the patency of IJV on preoperative and postoperative contrast-enhanced CT [57]. The incidence of internal jugular vein stenosis/occlusion in their study was 21.0%; interestingly all complete occlusion cases occurred on the left side and this observation was contributed to the lower pressure in the left IJV when compared to the right side. They concluded that postoperative radiotherapy and left-sided neck dissection were significant risk factors for occlusion [57]. Moreover, blindness, visual impairment, and ischemic optic neuropathy are rare but well-documented complications after bilateral or even unilateral radical neck dissection. The reason for blindness in most of the cases after radical neck dissection is optic neuropathy. Resection of internal jugular veins leads to increased intracranial pressure, with resultant decreased perfusion of the nerve [74–76].

The arterial complications associated with RND and MRND are mainly related to the involvement of the carotid artery by the tumor, which we will discuss in this chapter, and carotid blowout syndrome, which is presented in vascular complications in Chap. 7.

According to the American Joint Committee on Cancer (AJCC) – Cancer Staging, eighth edition, tumors with carotid involvement, invasion or encasement of the common or internal carotid artery, are staged as T4b. This situation is classified as stage IVB disease and is considered to be unresectable [58]. The most accepted definition of carotid artery encasement is defined as 270 degree or greater involvement of the carotid artery per radiographic imaging [59]. The classic study which reported this criterion was performed with MRI by Yousem et al. in 1995 [60]. However, based on the CT scan criteria, Yu et al. reported malignant tumor compression and deformation of the carotid artery of 180 degree or greater and undefined carotid artery wall, and fat or fascial plane deletion between the tumor and carotid artery should satisfy the criteria of carotid artery encasement [61].

The treatment of patients who have cervical metastasis involving the carotid artery has been controversial and challenging. The high risk of complications, loss of quality of life, and mortality must be balanced against the natural history of the disease if left untreated. Treatment options include radical surgical resection, chemoradiation, or palliative treatment; however, the prognosis of these patients is generally poor [63]. Roh et al. compared these treatment options and concluded that the survival benefit of aggressive radical surgery was not significantly greater than that of nonsurgical treatment methods [63]. However, aggressive treatment of disease involving the carotid artery may lead to better locoregional control of the disease [62].

Freeman et al. reported a series of 41 patients with an overall complication rate of 50%. The immediate postoperative mortality rate was 3%, the overall stroke rate was 20%, and the median survival was 12 months for patients dying of recurrent disease [62]. With the advancement of surgical interventions, the median survival for patients treated with surgery may be prolonged to 13.5 months compared with 3.6 months for patients treated with palliative intent [64]. Historically, the incidence of stroke during neck dissection was reported to be 3.2% and 4.8% [77, 78]. However, a recent review by Cramer et al. included 9697 patients, comparing 5827 patients who underwent head and neck surgery with neck dissection to 3870 patients who underwent major head neck surgery without neck dissection, and found the incidence of postoperative stroke to be 2.68% with bilateral neck dissection, 0.41% with unilateral neck dissection, and 0.24% without neck dissection. In their review, patients who had a history of carotid artery stenosis had an increased risk of postoperative stroke [79].

In general, carotid artery resection should be performed with the same oncologic surgical principles for advanced head and neck cancers and should be dictated by the aim for curative intent through en bloc resection with clear margins and acceptable morbidity and mortality risks. The decision to proceed with resection of the carotid artery is made during preoperative planning, not at the time of surgery [62]. There are three surgical approaches: (1) dissecting tumor from the involved carotid artery; (2) resecting the involved carotid artery together with the tumor and ligating the carotid artery without grafting; or (3) reconstructing the carotid artery at the time of arterial resection [65].

Dissection of the tumor off the carotid artery is advocated to minimize the postoperative complications, specifically cerebrovascular injuries [65]. Zhengang et al. reported a 62.5% recurrence rate when the tumor was dissected from the carotid artery compared to 59.6% when the carotid artery was resected. There was no statistical difference demonstrated in the survival rate between resecting the carotid artery and dissection of the tumor off the arterial wall [65]. Also, Kennedy et al. reported no significant differences in distant metastasis and neck recurrence rates when comparing carotid preservation with carotid resection [66]. However, dissection of cancer off the carotid artery does not provide an adequate surgical margin and weakens the carotid wall, predisposing it to rupture [62]. There is a high risk of incomplete resection, due to 40% having a microscopic invasion of the arterial wall by tumor cells [65]. Urken et al. suggested that carotid artery peel represents a non-oncological procedure [67]. However, if resection of the carotid artery is not possible because of unexpected involvement without preoperative cerebral perfusion studies or inability to reconstruct the artery in a patient lacking adequate collateral cerebral circulation, carotid "peel" may be beneficial [62].

Ligation of the carotid artery intraoperatively is associated with an unacceptable high rate of neurologic complications [62]. Moore et al. reported a comprehensive review and a series of 88 patients with carotid artery ligation. Forty patients (45.4%) developed cerebral complications and 27 patients (30.6%) died [68]. Stroke occurs immediately from an abrupt decrease in the cerebral blood flow or delayed blood flow caused by distal thrombus formation [62, 68]. The mechanism of injury appears to be thromboembolic, with late propagation of thrombus into an intracranial low-flow system [69]. To predict the possible postoperative neurological complications, the carotid stump pressure was evaluated in preoperative CT angiography and balloon occlusion test. Carotid stump pressures have been described as the best indicator for safe ligation of the carotid artery. If the stump pressure is >70 mmHg, there is little risk of impairment. If it is <50 mmHg, there is a high risk of cerebrovascular accidents. Even when the back pressure is >70 mmHg, so that adequate cerebral perfusion is maintained, patients are still at risk of thromboembolic complications [65].

Reconstruction of the carotid artery after resection is strongly recommended, even when a preoperative adequate cerebral collateral flow is documented [70]. The major advantages of carotid artery reconstruction are the preservation of ipsilateral cerebral blood flow and minimization of the risk of intraoperative stroke [65]. Recent studies have shown that carotid resection and reconstruction achieve acceptable neuromorbidities (5%) and mortalities (6.8%) when compared with carotid ligation morbidity of 17–45% and mortality of 8–58% reported in the literature [58].

Reconstruction of the carotid artery may be accomplished with the superficial femoral artery (SFA), saphenous vein, or polytetrafluoroethylene (PTFE) grafts. SFA grafts are durable and more resistant to infections than vein grafts but require reconstruction at the harvest site and thereby run risks of a conduit at a distant site and possible infection [71]. The saphenous vein is used more commonly by head neck surgeons to reconstruct the carotid with acceptable outcomes, mostly when it is covered with a myocutaneous flap [72]. The saphenous vein offers the advantage of resistance to infection; however, it is not resistant to tissue scarring and postoperative radiation therapy, which may cause fibrosis and graft occlusion or blowout. Furthermore, a mismatch between the saphenous vein and the carotid artery at anastomotic sites is not uncommon [73]. Polytetrafluoroethylene (PTFE) grafts have been used to reconstruct the carotid in uncontaminated fields and has led to the ability to perform aggressive en bloc resection of the carotid with one study citing excellent local control of the disease and survival [73].

Freeman et al. reported a protocol for the management of carotid artery resection. Preoperative clinical and radiographic examination of carotid artery involvement is crucial. The patient's collateral cerebral circulation was assessed through angiography. If patent carotid arteries and intact circle of Willis were demonstrated, a balloon-tipped catheter was inflated in the carotid (balloon test occlusion [BTO]) for 20 min, and the patient was monitored for any neurologic findings. After the temporary occlusion, technetium-99HMPAO was infused intravenously, and single photon emission computer tomography (SPECT) was performed. Any breakdown in the blood-brain barrier caused by ischemia was noted. After that, radical neck dissection and carotid resection are performed. Most of the patients had reconstruction with a saphenous vein graft if access to the superior and inferior portion of the carotid artery was possible. They also used a shunt and heparinization to maintain the blood flow while the carotid was resected with the neck contents. Finally, a pectoralis major myocutaneous flap was used for coverage [62].

Nerve Complications

In considering the complications of the radical and modified radical neck dissection in regard to neural structures, the potential nerves encountered are vast. The structures to be discussed include the spinal accessory nerve, the marginal mandibular branch of the facial nerve, vagus nerve, hypoglossal nerve, lingual nerve, and phrenic nerve.

Spinal Accessory Nerve

The spinal accessory nerve (SAN) should always be included in the discussion of potential complications of neck dissections because of its potentially profound impact on shoulder function. The SAN, cranial nerve XI, carries motor function innervating the sternocleidomastoid and the trapezius muscles. It follows a consistent course upon passing through the jugular foramen, where it follows the internal jugular vein closely. Most commonly, the nerve will course posteriorly and lateral to the internal jugular but can also be seen to course medially in a small subset of patients. It then emerges medially to the posterior belly of the digastric muscle, where it pierces the medial portion of the sternocleidomastoid muscle exiting the SCM posteriorly and entering the posterior triangle to ultimately reach the trapezius.

While many anatomical landmarks have been described for the reliable identification of the SAN, a commonly reported landmark is related to the general region where the cutaneous branches (lesser occipital, greater auricular, transverse cervical, and supraclavicular nerves) emerge into the subcutaneous tissues of the neck [80]. The SAN is typically described as being identifiable at a point 1–2 cm superior to this point. Many studies have mistakenly called this area Erb's point. Tubbs et al.

have described the difference between this point and the truly described Erb's point [80] located more inferiorly and related to the brachial plexus. A rough estimate for the entrance of the SAN to the SCM also corresponds with the junction of the upper and middle thirds of the SCM.

The original radical neck dissection was performed as an en bloc procedure, which included the sacrifice of the SAN among other non-lymphatic structures. Schuller et al. reported a prospective study of 50 radical neck dissection specimens, specifically exploring the potential for spinal accessory metastasis. Two relevant findings from this study are as follows: (1) 21 of the 28 neck specimens with metastasis had involvement of the jugular nodes with or without accessory nodal metastases and (2) seven of the neck specimens displayed isolated accessory nodal metastases (without any other cervical involvement) [81]. This paper from 1975 concluded that preservation of the SAN could not be justified [81]. While current management of the neck differs from Schuller's conclusions, this paper represents the eventual progression from the radical neck dissection to the conservative neck dissection, which has now become a mainstay in the management of the neck for head and neck oncology. The decision to preserve the SAN focuses on the benefits of postoperative shoulder function against the risk of incomplete resection of malignant disease along the accessory nodal chain. While there are no prospective trials comparing the radical neck dissection to a nerve-sparing dissection, there are various retrospective studies [82–84] examining this topic. While these studies suffer from many limitations that are inherent to retrospective studies, they nonetheless have established the oncologic safety in SAN-sparing dissections with comparable results to radical neck dissection. Brandenburg et al. evaluated 370 neck dissections for two series and found a 12% recurrence rate when the SAN was sacrificed and a 6% recurrence rate when the SAN was spared [82]. Skolnik et al. performed an anatomical study of 51 radical neck dissections and found that none of the specimens demonstrated metastasis in the posterior triangle. These authors suggested that the preservation of the posterior triangle was justified in the radical neck dissection [83]. Lastly, Bocca provides an anatomical explanation of the lymphatic structures of the neck and his 500 conservative neck dissections over 10 years. He describes a 2% recurrence rate, which follows the reported rates of recurrence with traditional radical neck dissections at the time of publication [84]. Ultimately, the presence of involved nodes or suspicious nodes along the path of the SAN is subject to the surgeon's clinical judgment for preservation or sacrifice.

The focus on SAN preservation versus sacrifice revolves around the profound disability that can occur from a constellation of symptoms referred to as "shoulder syndrome." The shoulder syndrome resulting from sacrifice during a radical neck dissection includes shoulder pain, limitation of abduction at the shoulder joint, full passive range of motion, and anatomical abnormalities consisting of a dropping of the affected shoulder [85]. Remmler et al. described a series of events initiated by sacrifice of the nerve resulting in a lateral descent of the scapula, which then translates into a down and forward drop of the shoulder. In addition to a cosmetic deformity, this leads to potential pain along the superior margin of the scapula, which is thought to be a result of recruitment of the levator scapulae and rhomboid muscles to compensate for the loss of trapezius function [86]. Preoperative patient counseling is important in setting expectations for both SAN-sacrificing and SAN-preserving neck dissections. Saunders et al. describe that 47% of patients who underwent SAN-preserving neck dissections displayed some degree of muscle atrophy and 20% showed little or no function of the muscle [87]. It is thus important to consider that a percentage of patients will show signs of SAN dysfunction even after preservation.

Various studies have been published examining the symptoms of patients with SAN-sacrificing neck dissection as well as the potential benefit of physical therapy [86, 88, 89]. Remmler et al. performed a prospective trial evaluating shoulder function after RND and MRND. Shoulder function was the primary outcome and was evaluated objectively by a physical therapist at various time points in the first year. Their results found that some patients within the SAN-sparing group had a temporary and reversible decrease in trapezius muscle function. This compared greatly to the patients in the SAN-sacrificing group who reported a profound and irreversible loss of function [86]. Sobol et al. addressed this same question by performing a prospective trial in 35 patients who underwent a total of 44 neck dissections. Outcomes included physical measurements of strength and range of motion, subjective perception of pain, and electromyography. They concluded that patients who underwent a modified radical neck dissection displayed clinically significant better shoulder function than the radical neck dissection group at 16 weeks. The critical difference between these two groups was found after 16 weeks, at which point the MRND group improved significantly compared to the RND group [88]. Schuller et al., on the other hand, describe a study involving questioning patients on the degree of permanent disability between MRND and RND groups. Interestingly, they found no reported difference in the complaint of numbness and no difference in return to work between the two groups [90].

In cases where the nerve has been sacrificed or injured, cable grafting has been studied as a reconstructive option for regaining shoulder function. Weisberger et al. studied 20 patients who underwent radical neck dissections with immediate reconstruction with cable grafting using the great auricular nerve. Shoulder function in the reconstructed group was better than patients who underwent radical neck dissections but worse than those who underwent a nerve-sparing neck dissection [91]. These studies and others emphasize the importance of these words quoted from Rogers et al.: "One should make every effort to preserve the SAN if it is not directly involved with tumor" [92].

Marginal Mandibular Branch of the Facial Nerve

The marginal mandibular branch carries motor function, which, when injured, can cause a significant functional and cosmetic deformity evidenced by asymmetry and dysfunctional movement of the lower lip. This can lead to deficits related to the management of saliva and swallowing difficulties related to lip incompetence.

The identification of the marginal mandibular branch of the facial nerve is a crucial part of the neck dissection procedure. After elevation of a subplatysmal flap, the marginal mandibular branch can be identified in an area spanning from the lateral portion of the mandible to 1 cm below the inferior border of the mandible. The marginal mandibular branch of the facial nerve is at greatest risk during dissection and removal of the level 1B nodal tissue. Of particular interest are the perifacial nodes as they should be included with the neck specimen and may also be intimately associated with the marginal mandibular branch of the facial nerve.

In non-oncologic surgeries, the Hayes Martin procedure is described as a safe dissection technique for protecting the marginal mandibular branch. After identifying the facial vein, it is ligated and cut. This then allows the elevation of the superficial layer of the deep cervical fascia from the submandibular gland in a superior direction. The marginal mandibular branch of the facial nerve will be included with the fascia resulting in the nerve being raised and rolled superiorly with the flap. This maneuver is a controversial dissection technique in neck dissections because it risks leaving undissected nodal tissue with the aim of minimizing dissection of the marginal mandibular branch of the facial nerve. Two conflicting studies have been published examining the safety of the Hayes Martin maneuver in neck dissections. Tierlli et al. completed a prospective study on 65 clinically negative neck specimens (49% oral cavity primary tumors) where the Hayes Martin maneuver was completed, and level 1B tissue was dissected. The fascial flap was then repositioned into its normal anatomical position, and dissection was carried out of the perifacial nodes hidden by the Hayes Martin maneuver. In this study, 84% of cases had perifacial nodes present that would have been missed by performing a Hayes Martin maneuver; the number of nodes ranged from 0 to 5 with a predominance of cases with two nodes. It is important to comment that clinically positive necks were excluded in this study.

Furthermore, this paper did not provide information on the incidence of perifacial nodal metastases. Given those caveats, the authors felt that the Hayes Martin maneuver was not an oncologically sound dissection technique given the risk of leaving potentially diseased nodal tissue [93]. The second study from Riffat et al. was a retrospective review of 34 patients (70% tonsil and posterior pharyngeal wall tumors) who had the Hayes Martin maneuver performed as part of the neck dissection. Median follow-up was 4 years, and no perifacial nodal regional recurrences were seen. The authors felt that the Hayes Martin maneuver was a safe oncologic procedure with the aim of protecting the marginal mandibular branch of the facial nerve [94]. Perifacial nodes are more commonly found to have metastatic disease in oral cavity squamous cell carcinoma as compared to oropharyngeal carcinoma. Given the large percentage of patients in this study that presented with oropharyngeal carcinoma, the perifacial nodes in this study's patient population may have represented an area of nodal tissue that was at lower risk for harboring metastatic disease.

The authors of this chapter favor the philosophy that a traditional Hayes Martin maneuver is not an oncologically sound dissection technique for neck dissections.

Fig. 7.3 Identification and
protection of the marginal
mandibular nerve

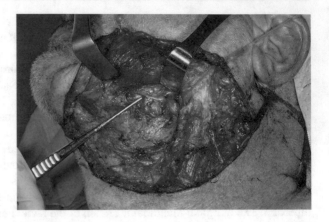

In our experience, by elevating a subplatysmal flap, the marginal mandibular branch
of the facial nerve will be located as described earlier: within a centimeter of the
inferior border of the mandible in the superficial layer of the deep cervical fascia.
By placing traction on the fascia, the nerve can sometimes be seen running in a horizontal direction. Once the nerve is identified, the fascia is incised, and the nerve is
dissected proximally and distally. If the nerve cannot be identified in this technique,
the facial vein can be identified, ligated, and cut as it courses over the lateral body
of the mandible. This reference point can then be used for careful dissection to identify the nerve. If found in this orientation, the nerve can be dissected proximally to
properly confirm the structure as the marginal mandibular branch of the facial nerve
(Fig. 7.3).

The lingual and the hypoglossal nerves are at risk in any form of neck dissection,
not only in RND and MRND. Injury to these nerves may result in loss of taste sensation, difficulty with speech, swallowing, and airway obstruction [95–98]. An attempt
should be made to preserve these nerves unless they display a clear evidence of
tumor involvement in which preservation would preclude appropriate oncologic
principles. Complications related to these nerves are discussed in a separate chapter.

Vagus Nerve

The vagus nerve, cranial nerve X, runs within the carotid sheath along with the
internal jugular vein and carotid artery. By dissecting the internal jugular vein cir-
cumferentially, the vagus nerve can be visualized throughout its course in the carotid
sheath. This is helpful in preventing inadvertent injury to the vagus nerve during
ligation of the internal jugular vein. Injury to the vagus nerve can manifest as
hoarseness, loss of sensation in the pharynx with resultant impaired cough protective mechanism, and possible chronic aspiration. There is a significant lack of
reported cases and an absence of studies related to outcomes after vagus nerve
injury. Li et al. reported a cases series of four patients who underwent lobectomy or
pneumonectomy with injury to the recurrent laryngeal nerve or vagus nerve with

immediate primary repair or cable grafting with the phrenic nerve. Overall, they reported success in the outcomes of speaking, lung infections, and dysphagia [142]. In the event of a vagus nerve transection, the surgeon should use his/her clinical judgment in the decision to perform or not perform a neurorrhaphy.

Phrenic Nerve

The phrenic nerve arises from the ventral rami of C3-C5 and travels inferiorly along the anterior surface of the anterior scalene muscle. Its function is related to the contraction of the ipsilateral diaphragm. In addition, it contains sensory and vasomotor fibers innervating the pericardium, the mediastinal and diaphragmatic pleura, and part of the parietal peritoneum [99]. Thus, many of the deficits that arise from injury to the phrenic nerve are related to loss of the natural ability to compensate for postoperative pulmonary changes. DeJong et al. conducted a retrospective study of 176 neck dissections and found unilateral phrenic nerve paralysis in 14 (8%) patients. Specifically, it was found that patients at higher risk for phrenic nerve paralysis included those who had fibrosis, edema, tumor infiltration in or near the phrenic nerve, or diffuse bleeding [99].

Infection

Wound infections in head and neck surgeries can be a result of many factors. While antibiotics play a large role in the reduction of wound infection, there are other patient-specific factors which affect the rate of infections as well. In discussing antibiotics, the nuances of route of administration, antibiotic type, duration, and dosages have been studied extensively in an effort to prevent wound infections. Postoperative infection rates can approach 100% in head and neck surgery without the use of perioperative parenteral antibiotics [100]. With the use of antibiotics, the overall rate of wound infection decreases to levels ranging from 8% to 25% [101–103].

The bacteriologic species that are present in head and neck surgery are specifically related to those commensal bacteria found within the upper aerodigestive tract. In the case of a clean operation, the typical commensal bacteria do not enter the surgical field. It is the clean-contaminated or dirty cases which pose a significantly increased risk of postoperative wound infections. The antibiotic coverage for an operation which enters the upper aerodigestive tract should provide appropriate coverage for *Eikenella corrodens*, Bacteroides sp., coagulase-negative *Staphylococcus*, *Streptococcus* sp., *Enterobacter* sp., *Fusobacterium*, and *Escherichia coli* [104]. Apart from considering the species of bacteria, the quantity of organisms is another major consideration. Becker et al. describe oropharyngeal secretions as containing large numbers of bacteria (10^{8-9}/ml) [105]. While colonization of a wound is not equivalent to wound infection, a bacterial load of 10^5/gram of tissue is often the quantity necessary to cause infection [104, 105].

Appropriate sterile technique and adequate irrigation after the completion of the procedure should be employed to reduce the bacterial load prior to closure.

In many of the reports in the literature about wound infection, there is a significant focus on identifying high-risk patients. Although many of these studies are retrospective, there are some trends and similarities that have been identified. Factors that have been evaluated include operative time, ASA staging, reconstruction method, blood replacement, placement of drains, concurrent tracheostomy, placement of nasogastric feeding tubes, and nutritional status. Cole et al. found that the infection rate in their cohort of patients was higher in the group of patients who underwent a surgery of >5 h duration compared to those between 4 and 5 h as well as those <4 h [106]. Nutritional status is also a factor that has been associated with wound infections. Larger tumors are more commonly found to cause impairments in the swallowing mechanism which can lead to malnutrition over time. This can lead to impaired wound healing which was found to have a correlation between wound infection and malnutrition by Robbins et al. [107]. Finally, wound infection was associated with radical or extended neck dissections with an OR of 14.61 compared to those undergoing less extensive neck dissections [108]. The extensive nature of the radical neck dissection, larger defect, and increased operative time lends itself to create an environment which can provide ample opportunities for bacterial overgrowth and wound infection [108].

T-staging has been found to be a risk factor for postoperative wound infection in various studies. Cole et al. examined 59 patients who underwent an oncologic head and neck clean-contaminated procedure and received cefazolin. Of these 59 patients, 67% of the infections were found to occur in T4 patients and 26% in T2/3 patients [106]. Man et al. studied 244 patients who underwent uncontaminated neck dissections. In this series of uncontaminated neck dissections, 3.3% of patients developed wound infections of which the majority of them underwent more extensive surgery for larger tumors [108]. Penel et al. studied tumor size in 165 clean contaminated procedures for squamous cell carcinoma of the upper aerodigestive tract. The wound infection rate was very high, 41%, representing an outlier in the literature for wound infections in patients who have received antibiotics. One possible explanation for the high rate of infections from the authors was that the majority (92/165) of the patients were staged with T3 or T4 tumors [109]. Alternatively, Girod et al. studied T staging related to complications and found that although higher T and N staging were found to have a tendency toward higher wound infections, these were not correlated with increased complications at a statistically significant value [103]. The correlation with N stage and infections is not as strong as with T stage. However, Robbins et al. did report a correlation between wound infections and N staging, where in 400 cases, a wound infection rate of 19.75% was found in patients with advanced nodal disease [107].

The benefit of preoperative parenteral antibiotics has been established in the literature as a cause of the significant drop in the incidence of wound infections after major head and neck procedures [110–113]. For further details, please refer to Chap. 3 on infectious complications of neck dissection.

Management of Recurrent Neck Disease

Despite adequate local control of Oral Squamous Cell Carcinoma (OSCC) and advances in treatment modality, recurrence rates of 25–48% have been reported [115]. Several studies have shown that recurrence after the initial treatment is most likely to occur in the first 24–36 months [114, 115]. Therefore, surveillance is important in the overall treatment of these patients [114, 115]. Treatment failure can be identified as persistent disease, local recurrence, regional recurrence, distant metastasis, and the development of a second primary tumor [114]. Locally persistent disease is defined as an incomplete response to definitive therapy or tumor that develops within 6 weeks of definitive therapy after a brief disease-free period. On the other hand, recurrent disease is defined as tumor that presents after a 6-week disease-free period [114]. Furthermore, recurrence can be further subdivided into recurrence at the tumor resection margins, local recurrence, recurrence in the neck, regional recurrence, and distant recurrence [114]. In this section, we will discuss the workup and the treatment options for the management of recurrent neck disease.

Workup and Diagnosis

Understanding that locoregional recurrences for head and neck malignancies can vary between 30% and 50% after definitive treatment [115, 122], the head and neck surgeon must be vigilant of recurrent disease, especially in the first 2 years. At the core of any surveillance regimen is the history and physical, including a complete head and neck exam as well as fiberoptic examination in appropriate cases where the oropharynx, hypopharynx, and glottis will require visualization. In cases where a suspicious lesion is found on clinical exam, the workup mirrors that of an initial malignant head and neck diagnosis. For lesions of the oral cavity or oropharynx which are easily accessible, a biopsy should be performed. For inaccessible lesions, the patient may require a panendoscopy under general anesthesia for adequate visualization and biopsy. For neck masses, a fine-needle aspiration may be pursued depending on the original pathology. Ultimately, a tissue biopsy is of paramount importance in determining treatment for recurrent neck disease [122].

Imaging is a significant adjunct in the workup of recurrent neck disease. CT scans of the soft tissues of the neck or MRI of the neck both offer excellent imaging modalities for recurrent disease. CT scans with contrast are equivalent to MRI when evaluating bony/cartilage erosion for oral cavity cancer, laryngeal cancer, and skull base lesions. MRI can provide more detailed information for bone marrow invasion of oral cavity cancers, nasopharyngeal cancers, sinonasal cancers, or any head and neck cancer where perineural tumor spread is of concern. FDG PET/CT in recurrent disease plays a larger role than in the initial presentation of malignant disease. FDG PET/CT has higher sensitivity for nodal and distant metastases over CT scans with contrast. Thus, patients with recurrent disease will typically undergo an FDG PET/CT to evaluate for nodal disease or distant metastases [122]. Krabbe et al. in prospective study evaluating the use of FDG PET/CT in the cancer surveillance and concluded that the [18] F-FDG PET is a suitable routine posttreatment surveillance tool in oral and oropharyngeal SCCa patients and detects malignancy before clinical suggestion by the regular follow-up arises. The best timing of a systematic [18] F-FDG PET scan is between 3 and 6 months after treatment [141].

Therapeutic strategies for recurrence in the neck remain a challenge and may vary widely from salvage surgery or reirradiation with curative intent to systemic therapies with a palliative aim, up to the choice not to perform any treatment for the progression of disease [4]. Furthermore, the managing multidisciplinary team should consider individual patient preferences, severity of symptoms, comorbidity burden, life expectancy, quality of life, toxicity of treatment, and its consequences in terms of surgical reconstruction or functional limitations [119].

Possible clinical situations of neck recurrence (NR) include neck recurrence after neck radiotherapy, NR after neck dissection, NR after combined therapy, NR in the untreated neck, NR with local recurrence (locoregional), NR with distant recurrence, NR with locoregional and distant recurrence, ipsilateral NR, contralateral NR, bilateral NR, and NR associated with tracheostomal recurrence [116]. The neck recurrence is challenging due to recurrent disease often found within the soft tissues of the neck rather than within the nodes that are surrounded by fibrofatty tissue [116]. Therefore, the treatment plan for these patients should be individualized, and the recommendation is generally offered on case by case basis.

Therapeutic strategies in the management of recurrent neck disease can be quite complex and depend primarily on the previous treatment and the extent of the disease at initial presentation [116]. Patients with neck recurrence without previous neck treatment generally undergo neck dissection with postoperative radiation therapy [5]. Tumors with disease involving the prevertebral fascia, skull base, encasing the carotid artery or great vessels in the mediastinum, and dermal invasion/metastasis are generally considered to be unresectable tumors [117]. Patients with distant metastases generally are not offered salvage surgery; however, in rare cases of isolated distant metastasis (e.g., an isolated lung metastasis) that can be definitively treated, salvage surgery may still be a reasonable option. Patients who have not been previously treated with radiation therapy will generally have better prognoses with surgical salvage, as postoperative radiation remains a more viable option [117]. Manzoor et al. reported that patients treated with a curative intent had a statistically better overall survival compared with the palliative group [64]. Furthermore, patients with previously untreated disease and those who underwent salvage surgery had a favorable prognosis compared with patients with recurrent or persistent disease. Previously untreated patients had a median overall survival of 38.7 months compared with a median overall survival of 9.6 months in patients with recurrent or persistent disease [64].

The National Comprehensive Cancer Network (NCCN) guidelines for Head and Neck Cancer [123] are used at our institution in guiding treatment of all malignant disease of the head and neck. With regard to recurrent neck disease, the three considerations that will heavily guide the recommended treatment include the presence of distant metastases, history of prior radiation therapy, and resectability of the recurrent disease. The NCCN guidelines prefer clinical trials when possible for those patients in whom there is controversy in management of their disease (e.g., reirradiation and unresectable disease) [123]. The guidelines are updated as clinical trial results are published that may provide a more advantageous treatment regimen [123].

Salvage Surgery

Before one decides what constitutes a radical procedure, it is necessary to bear in mind that very often the first treatment of cancer is an "all or nothing" affair. Either the growth is completely removed with all its metastases, or the patient's chance for life is either irrevocably lost or very seriously compromised. (Hayes Martin, 1961 [67])

The best chance for curing head and neck cancer is at the time of initial diagnosis. The outcomes of treatment of recurrent disease after prior definitive treatment are generally dismal [115]. Overall, 50% of the patients who present with recurrence in the neck are considered unsalvageable due to the advanced stage of the tumor at presentation, involvement of local vital structures, and poor surgical candidacy [115]. It is important to balance the potential for curing the patient with the inevitable significant decline in quality of life that occurs after salvage surgical treatment of recurrent tumors [115]. Aggressive surgical treatment is warranted when there is a significant chance of cure or durable palliation [115]. Patient selection is important to achieve acceptable outcomes; failure of salvage surgery for recurrent neck disease can lead to severe complications. A recurrent tumor in the neck may fungate through the skin or involves vital organs and structures, leading to considerable discomfort, ulceration, bleeding, and severe pain [116].

Salvage surgery is defined as surgery for recurrent or persistent disease after definitive cancer treatment has been previously performed [116]. Surgical salvage is often the only treatment option with curative intent for patients with recurrent neck disease [116]. Patients with recurrent SCCa from the oral cavity have an approximately 30–45% overall 5-year survival following salvage surgery [6]. However, there are several important prognostic factors that need to be considered by the managing multidisciplinary team prior to salvage surgery. These factors include the stage at recurrence and at the initial diagnosis, HPV status, site of the disease, disease-free interval, status of surgical margins, previous therapy, age, performance status, comorbidities, and patient desires and expectations [119].

To achieve a reasonable chance of cure by salvage surgery in recurrent neck disease, all margins should be clear from tumor. The utilization of either regional or free-flap reconstruction may offer the opportunity for a more aggressive resection and a better chance of achieving negative margins for potentially improved outcomes. However, wide margins remain difficult to obtain because of proximity to important structures, e.g., carotid artery [119]. Goodwin performed a meta-analysis of 32 studies with a total of 1080 patients (laryngeal 41%, pharyngeal 32%, oral cavity cancer 24%) and reported a 5-year survival rate of 39% after salvage surgery

[118]. The impact of the treated site was found to be less important than the stage of recurrence [118]. Patients with advanced recurrent tumors (rT3–4) and/or advanced recurrent nodal disease (rN2–3) have a poorer outcome as compared with patients with early-stage recurrence [119]. This is likely due to the difficulty in obtaining clear surgical margins in cases with higher T classification and by the higher risk of complications due to more extensive surgery [119]. Furthermore, a shorter disease-free interval predicts poorer outcome, as evidenced by several reports: generally, an interval of 6 months or less results in poorer patient outcome [119]. Positive margins or extracapsular spread has an increased risk for recurrence in primary as well as salvage surgery setting; some reports also show close margins as possible negative prognostic factors [119].

In patients who are treated with surgery alone, the incidence of recurrent disease in the neck was 30%, 50%, and 70% in N1, N2, and N3 neck diseases, respectively [116]. Therefore, the addition of radiotherapy after initial surgical treatment has increased over time to improve overall survival. Neck recurrence after surgery and radiotherapy is a challenging situation. Lim et al. reviewed 236 patients who developed a recurrence after primary curative surgery with or without radiation therapy for head and neck SCCA. They reported that the rate of isolated neck recurrence was 26% after primary surgical therapy and the overall salvage rate was 33% after salvage treatment [120]. Moreover, neck recurrence after surgery and chemoradiation was evaluated by Takashi et al. They evaluated salvage surgery for neck recurrence after surgery and chemoradiation and found that the 3-year overall survival after salvage surgery was 58.8% in the salvage surgery group and 8.59% in the other treatment group [118]. Luke et al. reviewed the outcomes of salvage surgery for neck recurrence for patients treated with primary concomitant chemoradiation [121]. They evaluated 204 patients – 38 patients underwent salvage surgery – and found that the 12- and 24-month overall survival rates were 60% and 27%, respectively.

In summary, salvage surgery with curative intent for recurrent neck disease without distant metastasis might be beneficial in small group of patients with favorable prognostic factors. The most critical aspect is patient selection and clinical judgment in determining which patients are appropriate candidates (Table 7.2).

Reirradiation

The possibility of incorporating reirradiation into a patient's treatment will rely strongly on appropriate patient selection. Those with no or insignificant comorbidity and toxicity of previous radiation therapy should be considered for reirradiation [124]. Standardized measurements and grading systems (Charlson comorbidity index, ACE-27, Karnofsky performance status, or ECOG performance scores) should be used. Dosage of previous radiation therapy, site of previous radiation therapy, recurrent tumor bulk, time from initial radiation therapy, and presence of neck disease should factor into the decision in reirradiating a patient [124]. While salvage surgery, when possible, provides a patient with the highest chance of cure, the need for reirradiation may be necessary with or without systemic therapy. It should be noted that clinical studies have been conducted which prove the

Table 7.2 Algorithm for the management of recurrent neck disease

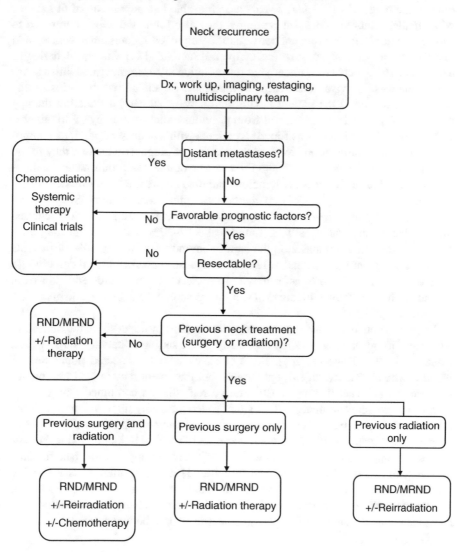

feasibility and efficacy of reirradiation using intensity-modulated radiation therapy (IMRT), 3D-radiation therapy, proton beam therapy, or stereotactic body radiation therapy [122].

In a systematic review, Strojan et al. discuss several key points related to reirradiation after salvage surgery; the same principles (adverse tumor features, margin status, nodal disease) that drive the need for adjunctive radiation in a primary malignancy should drive the need for reirradiation in a case of recurrent disease. Reirradiation comes with increased morbidity and mortality with more than a third of patients suffering grade 3 or 4 late toxicities and up to 8% of patients dying due to complications related to re-treatment. This review also found overall survival rates in the range of 40–50% at 2 years as achievable in a population of fit patients with smaller tumor volumes. Interestingly, they also found that when compared to salvage surgery alone, adjuvant reirradiation improves locoregional control and disease-free survival but has no effect on overall survival [124]. Choe et al. reviewed a cohort of 166 patients who underwent reirradiation in an attempt to establish prognostic factors of survival and treatment tolerance. Beneficial hazard ratios in this study were related to the patient having had salvage surgery, a radiation therapy dose of 60 Gy, and the time interval from previous radiation therapy of 36 months. A deleterious hazard ratio was found in patients with a history of previous chemoradiation. After stratification based on the number of prognostic factors, they found overall survival of 30% at 5 years in the most favorable risk group, whereas those with three to four unfavorable risk factors had died before the 5-year mark [127].

With regard to reirradiation in patients with unresectable tumors, Strojan et al. found that at 2 years, one-quarter to one-third of patients were free of locoregional tumor. Overall survival rates were found to be 10–30% at 2 years but long-term survivors were rare. Emphasizing the significant mortality, nearly 10% of patients will have treatment-related deaths [124]. The reconstruction of surgical defects with microvascular free tissue transfer may help protect vital structures and skin from reirradiation toxicity by reducing skin sloughing, spontaneous fistula, and great vessel rupture [128].

In cases where both reirradiation and systemic therapy are desired, the morbidity and mortality must be considered especially in the setting of salvage surgery (i.e., triple modality salvage therapy). Janot et al. evaluated a selected population of patients who all underwent salvage surgery but then were randomized into one of two groups: adjuvant therapy (postoperative reirradiation combined with chemotherapy) or no adjuvant therapy. This study found markedly improved locoregional control and disease-free survival in the adjuvant therapy group but no improvement in overall survival. The adjuvant therapy arm had a twofold reduction in local recurrences as compared with the group without adjuvant therapy, but this benefit came at a cost of increased acute and late toxicities [129]. Reirradiation is a feasible modality that has shown to improve locoregional control and disease-free survival in patients with recurrent disease. The morbidity and mortality of reirradiation are significant, and thus appropriate patient selection cannot be understated.

Systemic Therapy

For recurrent disease, systemic therapy plays a role when administered concurrently with reirradiation or as a palliative therapy. As a single modality, systemic therapy is used as palliation for patients with unresectable disease in whom reirradiation is contraindicated and salvage surgery is not possible. In addition, systemic therapy can be used for metastatic recurrent disease for palliation or prolongation of life. The decision to use combination systemic therapy or single-agent systemic therapy is a nuanced decision based on the patient's previous therapies and other patient-related factors (e.g., performance scores and comorbidities) [Fig. 7.4a,b].

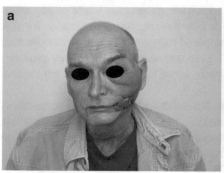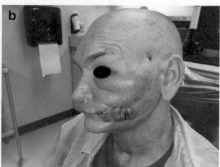

Fig 7.4 (**a** and **b**) Patient with recurrent SCCa of left buccal mucosa, left face, orbit, skull base and temporal bone, S/p primary CXRT. Stage IVB (rcT4bN1M0). Such patient might be a good candidate for systemic therapy

The EXTREME trial provides data that are cited within the NCCN guidelines for treatment of recurrent disease. This trial was a randomized phase III trial examining carboplatinum/cisplatin plus 5-flurouracil with or without the epidermal growth factor monoclonal antibody cetuximab. In the study arm in which cetuximab was added, median progression-free survival was prolonged from 3.3 to 5.6 months, as well as a prolongation in overall survival from 7.4 months to 10.1 months [130]. The second preferred regimen includes immunotherapy regimens that are currently undergoing clinical trials in the study of recurrent head and neck malignancies. Pembrolizumab, an anti-PD1 antibody [131], is one such immunotherapeutic agent that has shown improved overall survival in select patients. In considering patients for this therapy, an immunohistochemical assay is run on patient's tumor cells. The specimen is then given a "score" based on the results of the assay, which is termed the "Combined Positive Score" (CPS). Patients with PDL-1 CPS ≥ 20 and CPS ≥ 1 have shown an improved overall survival with the use of pemrolizumab [133, 134]. While single agent pembrolizumab can also be used in PDL-1 CPS ≥ 1, the NCCN recommendations do not make this a category 1 recommendation unless the CPS ≥ 20 [123, 132–134]. A phase 3 clinical trial comparing these two regimens (cetuximab/platinum/5-FU versus pembrolizumab/platinum/5-FU) has shown an overall survival advantage for patients treated with pembolizumab/platinum/5-FU as compared to cetuximab/platinum/5-FU [123, 134].

Ferris et al. reported a randomized phase III trial comparing an anti-PD1 antibody, nivolumab [131], to single agent systemic therapy (methotrexate, docetaxel, or cetuximab) with an improvement of overall survival. Importantly, the 1-year survival increased from 17% to 36% across the study arms [135, 136]. Nivolumab is recommended as an immunotherapy regimen for those patients with recurrent/metastatic disease which has progressed while on platinum-based therapy. A third immunotherapy agent, afatinib, was studied in a phase III trial comparing methotrexate in patients with recurrent disease who had progressed in spite of platinum-based therapy with some evidence of benefit to median progression-free survival in those patients whose tumors were HPV-negative, EGFR-amplified, HER3-low, and PTEN-high [137]. Afatinib is another immunotherapy that can be considered for patients with recurrent/metastatic disease which has progressed while on platinum-based therapy. It is important to distinguish that current recommendations for afatinib are based on lower-level evidence compared to pembrolizumab or nivolumab. Depending on patient-related factors and previous treatments, these three immunotherapies have proven efficacy in the treatment or palliation of patients with recurrent/metastatic disease.

Whether a patient undergoes traditional chemotherapy regimens or immunotherapy regimens, the overall survival on nonresectable recurrent disease remains low with a poor prognosis. The NCCN guidelines and authors of this chapter emphasize the importance of enrolling patients in clinical trials.

Palliative Care

While understanding that advances in surgery, radiation, and systemic therapy have improved our definitive and palliative management of recurrent disease, we acknowledge that the treatment is ultimately driven by the patients' wishes. Management of recurrent disease involves increased morbidity and mortality which the patient may not be willing to endure. As head and neck cancers can affect vital functions such as swallowing, speech, and breathing, it is important to remember that palliative care is a critical component of symptom management as the disease continues to progress. The majority of patients with head and neck cancer have advanced disease at the time of referral for palliative care, and many will die during their first admission to a palliative care unit [138]. The early and increased use of inpatient palliative care services allows for an improvement of symptom palliation over the traditional use of palliative care simply for management of death and complications [139]. By involving a palliative care team early, they can help guide treatment decision-making and support quality of life during and after treatment [140]. [Fig. 7.5a, b].

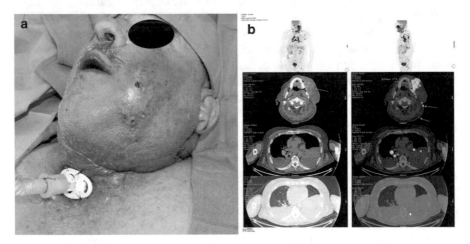

Fig 7.5 (**a** and **b**): Stage IVC (rcT4bN3bM1) SCCa of left buccal mucosa with distant metastases and dermal invasion. Tracheostomy and feeding tube to improve the palliative care

References

1. Patel KN, Shah JP. Neck dissection: past, present, future. Surg Oncol Clin N Am. 2005;14:461–77.
2. Ferlito A, Rinaldo A, et al. Neck dissection: past, present and future? The Journal of Laryngology & Otology. 2006;120:87–92.
3. Ferlito A, Rinaldo A, et al. Neck dissection: then and now. Auris Nasus Larynx. 2006;33:365–74.
4. Rinaldo A, Ferlito A, Silver CE. Early history of neck dissection. Eur Arch Otorhinolaryngol. 2008;265:1535–8.
5. Shaha AR. Radical neck dissection. Oper Tech Gen Surg. 2004;6(2):72–82.
6. Holmes JD. Neck dissection: nomenclature, classification, and technique. Oral Maxillofacial Surg Clin N Am. 2008;20:459–75.
7. Ferlito A, Rinaldo A, Robbins KT, et al. Changing concepts in the surgical management of the cervical node metastasis. Oral Oncol. 2003;39(5):429–35.
8. Myers EN, Fagan JJ. Treatment of the N þ neck in squamous cell carcinoma of the upper aerodigestive tract. Otolaryngol Clin N Am. 1998;31:671–86.
9. Jawdyn'ski F. Przypadek raka pierwotnego szyi. t.z. raka skrzelowego Volkmann'a.Wycie cie nowotworu wraz z rezekcyja te tnicy szyjowej wspo'lnej i z'yly szyjowej wewne trznej. Wyzdrowienie. Gaz Lek. 1888;8:530–7.
10. Towpik E. Centennial of the first description of the en bloc neck dissection. Plast Reconstr Surg. 1990;85:468–70.
11. Kierzek A. Otolaryngologia warszawska w kojcu XIX i na poczatku XX wieku. Otolaryngol Pol. 2003;57:761–4.
12. Crile GW. On the surgical treatment of cancer of the head and neckdwith a summary of one hundred and twenty-one operations performed upon one hundred and five patients. Trans South Surg Gynecol Assoc. 1905;18:108–27.
13. Crile GW. Excision of cancer of the head and neckdwith a special reference to the plan of dissection based on one hundred and thirty-two operations. JAMA. 1906;47:1780–6.
14. Martin HE, Del Valle B, Ehrlich H, et al. Neck dissection. Cancer. 1951;4:441–99.
15. Suárez O. El problema de las metastasis linfá ticas y alejadas del cá ncer de laringe e hipofaringe. Rev Otorrinolaringol. 1963;23:83–99.
16. Bocca EE. Evidement fonctionnel du cou dans la thérapie de principe de metastases ganglionnaires du cancer du larynx (Introduction à la présentation d'un film). J Fr Oto-rhinolaryngol. 1964;13:721–3.
17. Bocca E. Surgical management of supraglottic cancer and its lymph node metastases in a conservative perspective. Ann Otol Rhinol Laryngol. 1991;100:261–7.
18. Bocca E, Pignataro O, Oldini C, Cappa C. Functional neck dissection: an evaluation and review of 843 cases. Laryngoscope. 1984;94:942–5.
19. Bocca E, Pignataro O, Sasaki CT. Functional neck dissection. A description of operative technique. Arch Otolaryngol. 1980;106:524–7.
20. Bocca E, Pignataro O. A conservation technique in radical neck dissection. Ann Otol. 1967;76:975–87.
21. Bocca E. Supraglottic laryngectomy and functional neck dissection. J Laryngol Otol. 1966;80:831–6.
22. Gavila'n Alonso C, Blanco Galdı'n A, Sua'rez Nieto C. El vaciamiento funcional-radical cervicoganglionar. Anatomı'a quiru'rgica, te'cnica y resultados. Acta Otorinolaringol Ibero Am. 1972;23:703–817.
23. Gavila'n C, Gavila'n J. Five-year results of functional neck dissection for cancer of the larynx. Arch Otolaryngol Head Neck Surg. 1989;115:1193–6.
24. Gavila'n J, Gavila'n C, Herranz J. Functional neck dissection: three decades of controversy. Ann Otol Rhinol Laryngol. 1992;101:339–41.

25. Jesse RH, Ballantyne AJ, Larson D. Radical or modified neck dissection: a therapeutic dilemma. Am J Surg. 1978;136:516–9.
26. Gregor RT. Management of chyle fistulization in association with neck dissection. Otolaryngol Head Neck Surg. 2000;122(3):434e9.
27. Campisi CC, Boccardo F, Piazza C, Campisi C. Evolution of chylous fistula management after neck dissection. Curr Opin Otolaryngol Head Neck Surg. 2013;21:150–6.
28. Dedivitis RA, Guimarães AV, Pfuetzenreiter EG, Castro MA. Neck dissection complications. Braz J Otorhinolaryngol. 2011;77:65–9.
29. Crumley RL, Smith JD. Postoperative chylous fistula: prevention and management. Laryngoscope. 1976;86:804–13.
30. Roh JL, Yoon YH, Park CI. Chyle leakage in patients undergoing thyroidectomy plus central neck dissection for differentiated papillary thyroid carcinoma. Ann Surg Oncol. 2008;15:2576–80.
31. Dudic Y, Young L, McIntyre J. Neck dissection: past and present. Minerva Chir. 2010;65:45–58.
32. Yucel EA, et al. Evaluation of factors concerning the patency of the internal jugular vein after functional neck dissection. Eur Arch Otorhinolaryngol. 2003;260:35–8.
33. Williams PL, Warwick R, Dyson M, Bannister LH. Gray's Anatomy. 37th ed. Edinburgh: Churchill Livingstone; 1989.
34. Yucel EA, Orhan KS, Guldiken KY, Aydin K, Simsek T, Erdamar B, Deger K. Evaluation of factors concerning the patency of the internal jugular vein after functional neck dissection. Eur Arch Otorhinolaryngol. 2003;260:35–8. https://doi.org/10.1007/s00405-002-0517-3.
35. Downie SA, Schalop L, Mazurek JN, Savitch G, Lelonek GJ, Olson TR. Bilateral duplicated internal jugular veins: case study and literature review. Clin Anat. 2007;20:260–6.
36. Hashimoto Y, Otsuki N, Morimoto K, Saito M, Nibu K. Four cases of spinal accessory nerve passing through the fenestrated internal jugular vein. Surg Radiol Anat. 2012;34:373–5.
37. Moustafa Mourad MD, Masoud Saman MD, Yadranko Ducic MD. Internal to external jugular vein bypass allowing for simultaneous bilateral radical neck dissection. Laryngoscope. 2015;125:2480–4.
38. Leclerc G, Roy G. Le resection successive des deux jugulares internes au cours des evidements ganglionnaires bilateraux du cou. Presse Med. 1932;40:1382–3.
39. Dulguerov P, Soulier C, et al. Bilateral Radical Neck Dissection With Unilateral Internal Jugular Vein Reconstruction. Laryngoscope. 1998;108:1692–6.
40. Chae A, Sindelar WF. Bilateral radical neck dissection: report of results in 55 patients. Journal of Surgical Oncology. 1989;40:252–5.
41. Dulguervo P, Soulier C, Marurice J, Faidutti B, Allal A, Lehmann W. Bilateral radical neck dissection with unilateral internal jugular vein reconstruction. Laryngoscope. 1998;108:1692–6.
42. Weiss KL, Wax MK, Haydon RC, Kaufman HH, Hurst MK. Intracranial pressure changes during bilateral radical neck dissections. Head Neck. 1993;15:546–52.
43. Sugarbaker E, Wiley H. Intracranial pressure studies incident to resection of the internal jugular veins. Cancer. 1951;4:242–50.
44. Milner G. Case of blindness after bilateral neck dissection. J Laryngol Otol. 1960;74:880–5.
45. Torti RA, Ballantyne AJ, Berkeley RG. Sudden blindness after simultaneous bilateral radical neck dissection. Arch Surg. 1964;88:271–4.
46. McQuarrie DG, Mayberg M, Ferguson M, Schons AR. A physiologic approach to the problems of simultaneous bilateral neck dissection. Am J Surg. 1977;134:455–60.
47. Wenig BL, Heller KS. The syndrome of inappropriate secretion of antidiuretic hormone (SIADH) following neck dissection. Laryngoscope. 1984;97:467–70.
48. Razack M, Baffi R, Sako K. Bilateral radical neck dissection. Cancer. 1981;47:199.
49. McGuirt WF Sr, BF MC. Bilatseral radical neck dissections. Arch Otolaryngology. 1980;106:427–9.
50. Ward MJA, Faris C, Upile T, Patel NN. Ophthalmoplegia secondary to raised intracranial pressure after unilateral neck dissection with internal jugular vein sacrifice. Head Neck. 2011;33:587–90. https://doi.org/10.1002/hed.21309.

51. Doepp F, Hoffmann O, Schreiber S, Lammert I, Einhaupl KM, Valdueza JM. Venous collateral blood flow assessed by Doppler ultra- sound after unilateral radical neck dissection. Ann Otol Rhinol Laryngol. 2001;110:893–906.
52. Gius JA, Grier DH. Venous adaptation following bilateral radical neck dissection with excision of the jugular veins. Surgery. 1950;28:1503–8.
53. Kamizono, et al. Internal jugular vein reconstruction: application of conventional type a and novel type K methods. The Journal of Laryngology & Otology. 2011;125:643–8.
54. Katsuno S, et al. Three types of internal jugular vein reconstruction in bilateral radical neck dissection. Laryngoscope. September 2000;110:1578–80.
55. Fisher CB, Mattox DE, Zinreich JS. Patency of the internal jugular vein after functional neck dissection. Laryngoscope. 1988;98:923–7.
56. Makiguchi T, Yokoo S, Ogawa M, Miyazaki H. Factors influencing internal jugular vein patency after neck dissection in oral cancer. Int J Oral Maxillofac Surg. 2015;44:1218–24.
57. Ozer E, Agrawal A, Ozer HG, Schuller DE. The impact of surgery in the management of the head and neck carcinoma involving the carotid artery. Laryngoscope. 2008;118(10):1771–4.
58. Krol E, et al. Vascular interventions in head and neck cancer patients as a marker of poor survival. J Vasc Surg. 2019;69:181–9.
59. Yousem DM, Hatabu H, Hurst RW, et al. Carotid artery invasion by head and neck masses: prediction with MR imaging. Radiology. 1995;195(3):715–20.
60. Yu Q, et al. Carotid artery and jugular vein invasion of oral-maxillofacial and neck malignant tumors: diagnostic value of computed tomography. Oral Surg Oral Med Oral Pathol Oral Radiol Endod. 2003;96:368–72.
61. Freeman SB, Hamaker RC, Borrowdale RB, Huntley TC. Management of neck metastasis with carotid artery involvement. Laryngoscope. 2004;114:20–4.
62. Roh J-L, Kim MR, Choi S-H, et al. Can patients with head and neck cancers invading carotid artery gain survival benefit from surgery?
63. Manzoor NF, Russell JO, Bricker A, et al. Impact of surgical resection on survival in patients with advanced head and neck cancer involving the carotid artery. JAMA Otolaryngol Head Neck Surg. 2013;139:1219e25.
64. Roh J-L, Kim MR, Choi S-H, et al. Can patients with head and neck cancers invading carotid artery gain survival benefit from surgery?. Acta Otolaryngol. 2008;128:1370–4.
65. Kennedy JT, Krause CJ, Loevy S. The importance of tumor attachment to the carotid artery. Arch Otolaryngol. 1977;103:70–3.
66. Urken M, Biller HF, Lawson W. Salvage surgery for recurrent neck carcinoma after multimodality therapy. Head Neck Surg. 1986;8:332–42.
67. Moore OS, Baker HW. Carotid artery ligation in surgery of the head and neck. Cancer. 1955;8:712.
68. Ehrenfeld WK, Stone RJ, Wylie EJ. Relation of carotid stump pressure to safety of carotid artery ligation. Surgery. 1983;93:299–305.
69. Meleca RJ, Marks SC. Carotid artery resection for cancer of the head and neck. Arch Otolaryngol Head Neck Surg. 1994;120:974–8.
70. Guo Y, Pang MC-Y, Teo CE-H, Chng JK. Carotid artery involvement in advanced recurrent head and neck cancer: a case report and literature review. Ann Vasc Surg. 2019;56:355.e11–5.
71. McCready RA, Miller SK, Hamaker RC, et al. What is the role of carotid arterial resection in the management of advanced cervical cancer? J Vasc Surg. 1989;10:274e80.
72. Giulio Illuminati MD, Fabrice Schneider MD, Antonio Minni MD, Francesco G, Calio MD, Giulia Pizzardi MD, Jean-Baptiste Ricco MD. Resection of recurrent neck cancer with carotid artery replacement. J Vasc Surg. 2016;63:1272–8.
73. Aydin O, Memisoglu I, Ozturk M, Altintas O. Anterior ischemic optic neuropathy after unilateral radical nec dissection: case report and review. Auris Nasus Larynx. 2008;35:308–12.
74. Pazos GA, Leonard DW, Blice J. Blindness after bilateral neck dissection: case report and review. Am J Otolaryngol. 1999;20:340–5.
75. Marks SC, Jacques DA, Hirata RM. Blindness following bilateral radical neck dissection. Head Neck. 1990;12:342–5.

76. Thompson SK, Southern DA, McKinnon JG, et al. Incidence of perioperative stroke after neck dissection for head and neck cancer: a regional outcome analysis. Ann Surg. 2004;239:428–31.

77. Nosan DK, Gomez CR, Maves MD. Perioperative stroke in patients undergoing head and neck surgery. Ann Otol Rhinol Laryngol. 1993;102:717–23.

78. John D. Cramer, Patel UA, Maas MB, Samant S, Smith SS. Is neck dissection associated with an increased risk of postoperative stroke? Otolaryngology – Head and Neck Surgery. 2017;157(2):226–32.

79. Tubbs RS, Loukas M, Salter EG, Oakes WJ, Erb W. Wilhelm Erb and Erb's point. Clin Anat. 2007 Jul;20(5):486–8. https://doi.org/10.1002/ca.20385.

80. Schuller DE, Platz CE, Krause CJ. Spinal accessory lymph nodes: a prospective study of metastatic involvement. Laryngoscope. 1978 Mar;88(3):439–50. https://doi.org/10.1288/00005537-197803000-00008.

81. Brandenburg JH, Lee CY. The eleventh nerve in radical neck surgery. Laryngoscope. 1981 Nov;91(11):1851–9. https://doi.org/10.1288/00005537-198111000-00009.

82. Skolnik EM, Yee KF, Friedman M, Golden TA. The posterior triangle in radical neck surgery. Arch Otolaryngol. 1976 Jan;102(1):1–4. https://doi.org/10.1001/archotol.1976.00780060047002.

83. Bocca E. Conservative neck dissection. Laryngoscope. 1975 Sep;85(9):1511–5. https://doi.org/10.1288/00005537-197509000-00013.

84. Nahum AM, Mullally W, Marmor L. A syndrome resulting from radical neck dissection. Arch Otolaryngol. 1961 Oct;74:424–8. https://doi.org/10.1001/archotol.1961.00740030433011.

85. Remmler D, Byers R, Scheetz J, Shell B, White G, Zimmerman S, et al. A prospective study of shoulder disability resulting from radical and modified neck dissections. Head Neck Surg. 1986 Mar-Apr;8(4):280–6. https://doi.org/10.1002/hed.2890080408.

86. Saunders JR, Hirata RM, Jaques DA. Considering the spinal accessory nerve in head and neck surgery. Am J Surg. 1985 Oct;150(4):491–4. https://doi.org/10.1016/0002-9610(85)90161-8.

87. Sobol S, Jensen C, Sawyer W, Costiloe P, Thong N. Objective comparison of physical dysfunction after neck dissection. Am J Surg. 1985 Oct;150(4):503–9. https://doi.org/10.1016/0002-9610(85)90164-3.

88. Kuntz AL, Weymuller EA. Impact of neck dissection on quality of life. Laryngoscope. 1999 Aug;109(8):1334–8. https://doi.org/10.1097/00005537-199908000-00030.

89. Schuller DE, Reiches NA, Hamaker RC, Lingeman RE, Weisberger EC, Suen JY, et al. Analysis of disability resulting from treatment including radical neck dissection or modified neck dissection. Head Neck Surg. 1983 Sep-Oct;6(1):551–8. https://doi.org/10.1002/hed.2890060103.

90. Weisberger EC, Kincaid J, Riteris J. Cable grafting of the spinal accessory nerve after radical neck dissection. Arch Otolaryngol Head Neck Surg. 1998 Apr;124(4):377–80. https://doi.org/10.1001/archotol.124.4.377.

91. Rogers SN, Ferlito A, Pellitteri PK, Shaha AR, Rinaldo A. Quality of life following neck dissections. Acta Otolaryngol. 2004 Apr;124(3):231–6. https://doi.org/10.1080/00016480310015317.

92. Tirelli G, Marcuzzo AV. Lymph nodes of the perimandibular area and the hazard of the hayes martin maneuver in neck dissection. Otolaryngol Head Neck Surg. 2018;159(4):692–7. https://doi.org/10.1177/0194599818773084.

93. Riffat F, Buchanan MA, Mahrous AK, Fish BM, Jani P. Oncological safety of the Hayes-Martin manoeuvre in neck dissections for node-positive oropharyngeal squamous cell carcinoma. J Laryngol Otol. 2012 Oct;126(10):1045–8. https://doi.org/10.1017/S0022215112001740.

94. Bageant TE, Tondini D, Lysons D. Bilateral hypoglossal-nerve palsy following a second carotid endarterectomy. Anesthesiology. 1975 Nov;43(5):595–6. https://doi.org/10.1097/00000542-197511000-00026.

95. Dehn TC, Taylor GW. Cranial and cervical nerve damage associated with carotid endarterectomy. Br J Surg. 1983 Jun;70(6):365–8. https://doi.org/10.1002/bjs.1800700619.

96. Swift TR. Involvement of peripheral nerves in radical neck dissection. Am J Surg. 1970 Jun;119(6):694–8. https://doi.org/10.1016/0002-9610(70)90241-2.
97. Keane JR. Twelfth-nerve palsy. Analysis of 100 cases. Arch Neurol. 1996 Jun;53(6):561–6. https://doi.org/10.1001/archneur.1996.00550060105023.
98. de Jong AA, Manni JJ. Phrenic nerve paralysis following neck dissection. Eur Arch Otorhinolaryngol. 1991;248(3):132–4. https://doi.org/10.1007/BF00178921.
99. Grandis JR, Vickers RM, Rihs JD, Yu VL, Wagner RL, Kachman KK, et al. The efficacy of topical antibiotic prophylaxis for contaminated head and neck surgery. Laryngoscope. 1994 Jun;104(6 Pt 1):719–24. https://doi.org/10.1288/00005537-199406000-00011.
100. Cole RR, Robbins KT, Cohen JI, Wolf PF. A predictive model for wound sepsis in oncologic surgery of the head and neck. Otolaryngol Head Neck Surg. 1987 Feb;96(2):165–71. https://doi.org/10.1177/019459988709600209.
101. Brown BM, Johnson JT, Wagner RL. Etiologic factors in head and neck wound infections. Laryngoscope. 1987 May;97(5):587–90. https://doi.org/10.1288/00005537-198705000-00009.
102. Girod DA, McCulloch TM, Tsue TT, Weymuller EA. Risk factors for complications in clean-contaminated head and neck surgical procedures. Head Neck. 1995 Jan-Feb;17(1):7–13. https://doi.org/10.1002/hed.2880170103.
103. Kim DD, Ord RA. Complications in the treatment of head and neck cancer. Oral Maxillofac Surg Clin North Am. 2003 May;15(2):213–27. https://doi.org/10.1016/S1042-3699(02)00100-0.
104. Becker GD. Identification and management of the patient at high risk for wound infection. Head Neck Surg. 1986 Jan-Feb;8(3):205–10. https://doi.org/10.1002/hed.2890080313.
105. Robbins KT, Favrot S, Hanna D, Cole R. Risk of wound infection in patients with head and neck cancer. Head Neck. 1990 Mar-Apr;12(2):143–8. https://doi.org/10.1002/hed.2880120209.
106. Man LX, Beswick DM, Johnson JT. Antibiotic prophylaxis in uncontaminated neck dissection. Laryngoscope. 2011 Jul;121(7):1473–7. https://doi.org/10.1002/lary.21815.
107. Penel N, Lefebvre D, Fournier C, Sarini J, Kara A, Lefebvre JL. Risk factors for wound infection in head and neck cancer surgery: a prospective study. Head Neck. 2001 Jun;23(6):447–55. https://doi.org/10.1002/hed.1058.
108. Weber RS, Raad I, Frankenthaler R, Hankins P, Byers RM, Guillamondegui O, et al. Ampicillin-sulbactam vs clindamycin in head and neck oncologic surgery. The need for gram-negative coverage. Arch Otolaryngol Head Neck Surg. 1992 Nov;118(11):1159–63. https://doi.org/10.1001/archotol.1992.01880110027007.
109. Mitchell RM, Mendez E, Schmitt NC, Bhrany AD, Futran ND. Antibiotic prophylaxis in patients undergoing head and neck free flap reconstruction. JAMA Otolaryngol Head Neck Surg. 2015 Dec;141(12):1096–103. https://doi.org/10.1001/jamaoto.2015.0513.
110. Balamohan SM, Sawhney R, Lang DM, Cherabuddi K, Varadarajan VV, Bernard SH, et al. Prophylactic antibiotics in head and neck free flap surgery: a novel protocol put to the test. Am J Otolaryngol. 2019;40(6):102276. https://doi.org/10.1016/j.amjoto.2019.102276.
111. Simons JP, Johnson JT, Yu VL, Vickers RM, Gooding WE, Myers EN, et al. The role of topical antibiotic prophylaxis in patients undergoing contaminated head and neck surgery with flap reconstruction. Laryngoscope. 2001 Feb;111(2):329–35. https://doi.org/10.1097/00005537-200102000-00026.
112. Petrisor D, Fernandes R. Reoperative maxillofacial oncology. Oral Maxillofacial Surg Clin N Am. 2011;23:161–8.
113. Kademani D, Dierks E. Management of locoregional recurrence in oral squamous cell carcinoma. Oral Maxillofacial Surg Clin N Am. 2006;18:615–25.
114. Takashi, et al. Comparison of salvage surgery for recurrent or residual head and neck squamous cell carcinoma. Jpn J Clin Oncol. 2019:1–9.
115. Bossi P, et al. Prognostic and predictive factors in recurrent and/or metastatic head and neck squamous cell carcinoma: a review of the literature. Critical Reviews in Oncology / Hematology. 2019;137:84–91.

116. Maruo T, Zenda S, Shinozaki T, Tomioka T, Okano W, Sakuraba M, Tahara M, Hayashi R. Comparison of salvage surgery for recurrent or residual head and neck squamous cell carcinoma. Jpn J Clin Oncol. 2020 Mar 9;50(3):288-295. doi: 10.1093/jjco/hyz176. PMID: 31845736.
117. Zafereo M. Surgical salvage of recurrent cancer of the head and neck. Curr Oncol Rep. 2014;16:386.
118. Goodwin WJ Jr. Salvage surgery for patients with recurrent squamous cell carcinoma of the upper aerodigestive tract: when do the ends justify the means? Laryngoscope. 2000;(3 Pt. 2 Suppl. 93):110, 1–8.
119. Zafereo ME, Hanasono MM, Rosenthal DI, et al. The role of salvage surgery in patients with recurrent squamous cell carcinoma of the oropharynx. Cancer. 2009;115(24):5723–33.
120. Lim JY, Lim YC, Kim SH, et al. Factors predictive of successful outcome following salvage treatment of isolated neck recurrences. Otolaryngol Head Neck Surg. 2010;142(6):832–7.
121. Richey L, Shores CG, Georage J, et al. The effectiveness of salvage surgery after the failure of primary concomitant chemoradiation in head and neck cancer. Otolaryngol Head Neck Surg. 2007;136:98–103.
122. Takiar V, Garden AS, Ma D, Morrison WH, Edson M, Zafereo ME, et al. Reirradiation of head and neck cancers with intensity modulated radiation therapy: outcomes and analyses. Int J Radiat Oncol Biol Phys. 2016;95(4):1117–31. https://doi.org/10.1016/j.ijrobp.2016.03.015.
123. National Comprehensive Cancer Network: clinical practice guidelines in oncology. https://www.nccn.org/professionals/physician_gls/pdf/head-and-neck.pdf (2019). Accessed 05 Apr 2020.
124. Strojan P, Corry J, Eisbruch A, Vermorken JB, Mendenhall WM, Lee AW, et al. Recurrent and second primary squamous cell carcinoma of the head and neck: when and how to reirradiate. Head Neck. 2015 Jan;37(1):134–50. https://doi.org/10.1002/hed.23542.
125. Romesser PB, Cahlon O, Scher ED, Hug EB, Sine K, DeSelm C, et al. Proton beam Reirradiation for recurrent head and neck Cancer: multi-institutional report on feasibility and early outcomes. Int J Radiat Oncol Biol Phys. 2016 May 1;95(1):386–95. https://doi.org/10.1016/j.ijrobp.2016.02.036.
126. Phan J, Sio TT, Nguyen TP, Takiar V, Gunn GB, Garden AS, et al. Reirradiation of head and neck cancers with proton therapy: outcomes and analyses. Int J Radiat Oncol Biol Phys. 2016;96(1):30–41. https://doi.org/10.1016/j.ijrobp.2016.03.053.
127. Choe KS, Haraf DJ, Solanki A, Cohen EE, Seiwert TY, Stenson KM, et al. Prior chemoradiotherapy adversely impacts outcomes of recurrent and second primary head and neck cancer treated with concurrent chemotherapy and reirradiation. Cancer. 2011 Oct 15;117(20):4671–8. https://doi.org/10.1002/cncr.26084.
128. Suh JD, Kim BP, Abemayor E, Sercarz JA, Nabili V, Liu JH, et al. Reirradiation after salvage surgery and microvascular free flap reconstruction for recurrent head and neck carcinoma. Otolaryngol Head Neck Surg. 2008 Dec;139(6):781–6. https://doi.org/10.1016/j.otohns.2008.09.002.
129. Janot F, de Raucourt D, Benhamou E, Ferron C, Dolivet G, Bensadoun RJ, et al. Randomized trial of postoperative reirradiation combined with chemotherapy after salvage surgery compared with salvage surgery alone in head and neck carcinoma. J Clin Oncol. 2008 Dec 1;26(34):5518–23. https://doi.org/10.1200/JCO.2007.15.0102.
130. Vermorken JB, Mesia R, Rivera F, Remenar E, Kawecki A, Rottey S, et al. Platinum-based chemotherapy plus cetuximab in head and neck cancer. N Engl J Med. 2008 Sep 11;359(11):1116–27. https://doi.org/10.1056/NEJMoa0802656.
131. Sim F, Leidner R, Bell RB. Immunotherapy for head and neck Cancer. Oral Maxillofac Surg Clin North Am. 2019 Feb;31(1):85–100. https://doi.org/10.1016/j.coms.2018.09.002.
132. Cohen EEW, Soulières D, Le Tourneau C, Dinis J, Licitra L, Ahn MJ, et al. Pembrolizumab versus methotrexate, docetaxel, or cetuximab for recurrent or metastatic head-and-neck squamous cell carcinoma (KEYNOTE-040): a randomised, open-label, phase 3 study. Lancet. 2019;393(10167):156–67. https://doi.org/10.1016/S0140-6736(18)31999-8.

133. Burtness B, Harrington KJ, Greil R. KEYNOTE-048: phase 3 study of first-line pembroli-zumab (P) for recurrent/metastatic head and neck squamous cell carcinoma (R/M HNSCC). https://oncologypro.esmo.org/meeting-resources/esmo-2018-congress/KEYNOTE-048-Phase-3-study-of-first-line-pembrolizumab-P-for-recurrent-metastatic-head-and-neck-squamous-cell-carcinoma-R-M-HNSCC. Accessed 15 Apr 2020.

134. Rischin D, Harrington KJ, Greil R. Protocol-specified final analysis of the phase 3 KEYNOTE-048 trial of pembrolizumab (pembro) as first-line therapy for recurrent/ meta-static head and neck squamous cell carcinoma (R/M HNSCC). J Clin Oncol. 2019;37(15_suppl) Abstract 6000

135. Ferris RL, Blumenschein G, Fayette J, Guigay J, Colevas AD, Licitra L, et al. Nivolumab for recurrent squamous-cell carcinoma of the head and neck. N Engl J Med. 2016;375(19):1856–67. https://doi.org/10.1056/NEJMoa1602252.

136. Harrington KJ, Ferris RL, Blumenschein G, Colevas AD, Fayette J, Licitra L, et al. Nivolumab versus standard, single-agent therapy of investigator's choice in recurrent or metastatic squa-mous cell carcinoma of the head and neck (CheckMate 141): health-related quality-of-life results from a randomised, phase 3 trial. Lancet Oncol. 2017;18(8):1104–15. https://doi.org/10.1016/S1470-2045(17)30421-7.

137. Machiels JP, Haddad RI, Fayette J, Licitra LF, Tahara M, Vermorken JB, et al. Afatinib versus methotrexate as second-line treatment in patients with recurrent or metastatic squamous-cell carcinoma of the head and neck progressing on or after platinum-based therapy (LUX-Head & Neck 1): an open-label, randomised phase 3 trial. Lancet Oncol. 2015 May;16(5):583–94. https://doi.org/10.1016/S1470-2045(15)70124-5.

138. Forbes K. Palliative care in patients with cancer of the head and neck. Clin Otolaryngol Allied Sci. 1997 Apr;22(2):117–22. https://doi.org/10.1046/j.1365-2273.1997.00872.x.

139. Mulvey CL, Smith TJ, Gourin CG. Use of inpatient palliative care services in patients with metastatic incurable head and neck cancer. Head Neck. 2016 Mar;38(3):355–63. https://doi.org/10.1002/hed.23895.

140. McCammon SD. Concurrent palliative care in the surgical management of head and neck cancer. J Surg Oncol. 2019 Jul;120(1):78–84. https://doi.org/10.1002/jso.25452.

141. Krabbe CA, Pruim J, Dijkstra PU, et al. 18F-FDG PET for routine posttreatment surveillance in oral and oropharyngeal squamous cell carcinoma. J Nucl Med. 2010;51:1164–5.

142. Li H, Hu Y, Huang J, Yang Y, Xing K, Luo Q. Attempt of peripheral nerve reconstruction during lung cancer surgery. Thorac Cancer. 2018;9(5):580–3.

143. George K. Surgical techniques for parotid and submandibular glands and Ranulae. In: Brennan P, Schliephake H, Ghali GE, Cascarini L, editors. Maxillofacial surgery. St. Louis: Elsevier; 2017. p. 686–9.

Other Complications Related to Neck Dissection

8

Roderick Y. Kim, Todd R. Wentland, Daniel A. Hammer, and Fayette C. Williams

Introduction

Throughout this textbook, we discussed well-described and more frequently observed complications of neck dissections. However, with time, most surgeons with an active practice will experience the "zebras." This chapter aims to shed light on these less frequent complications that reasonably will occur during the span of an oral, head, and neck surgeon's career with review of the literature, where available.

Preoperative Considerations

The old adage says, "An ounce of prevention is worth a pound of cure," rings especially true when discussing uncommon complications in neck dissection. These complications are rarely controlled with the knife, cautery, or suture. In contrast, these complications require foresight to identify the potential causative factors and implement preventative strategies to mitigate the risk to the patient. This process begins during the patient's first clinic visit and initial history and physical examination, with the goal of optimizing the patient's medical comorbidities prior to surgical intervention. This approach recognizes that there are significant factors in the

R. Y. Kim (✉) · F. C. Williams
John Peter Smith Health Network, Department of Oral and Maxillofacial Surgery, Division of Maxillofacial Oncology and Reconstructive Surgery, Fort Worth, TX, USA

Department of Surgery, Texas Christian University, Fort Worth, TX, USA
e-mail: rkim01@jpshealth.org

T. R. Wentland · D. A. Hammer
John Peter Smith Health Network, Department of Oral and Maxillofacial Surgery, Division of Maxillofacial Oncology and Reconstructive Surgery, Fort Worth, TX, USA

© Springer Nature Switzerland AG 2021
T. Schlieve, W. Zaid (eds.), *Complications in Neck Dissection*,
https://doi.org/10.1007/978-3-030-62739-3_8

preoperative setting that have a direct impact on patient outcomes regardless of the surgeon's experience level and surgical expertise.

Surgical quality improvement has gained significant attention, and this is high-lighted by the creation of the American College of Surgeons Nation Surgical Quality Improvement Program® (NISQIP®), which "aims to zero in on preventable com-plications" (https://www.facs.org/quality-programs/acs-nsqip). NSQIP was devel-oped in the 1990s by the Veterans Affairs system for general and vascular surgery. The NSQIP was soon widely accepted after demonstrating a 45% reduction in post-operative morbidity and a 27% decline in postoperative mortality by recognizing at-risk patient factors prior to surgery and addressing them preoperatively [1]. Although proven to be successful in general surgery, until 2016, there was no head and neck specific risk-stratification tool within NSQIP. Head and neck surgical patients are unique in that their surgical interventions may directly impact so many of the attributes that make us human, such as speech and swallow function. These functional outcomes and the use of feeding tubes and tracheostomy tubes are not included in the NSQIP. In addition, it has been demonstrated that the Surgical Risk Calculator (SRC) of the NSQIP is a poor predictor for surgical outcome among patients undergoing microvascular head and neck reconstruction, which is very common in head and neck surgery today [2].

In response to the shortcomings of the NSQIP for head and neck surgery, Lewis et al. developed and validated the Head and Neck-Reconstructive Surgery NSQIP [3]. The preoperative variables identified that impact long-term patient outcomes are not surprising: tobacco pack-years, alcohol abuse prior to surgery, presence of feeding tube, degree of dependence on feeding tube, presence of tracheostomy tube, TNM stage, anatomical subsite of disease, previous chemotherapy or radiation, and previous local and/or regional disease. Of all these considered factors on patient outcomes, only current smoking, current alcohol abuse, and hypertension requiring medication were statistically significant and correlated to serious postoperative morbidity defined as cardiac arrest requiring cardiopulmonary resuscitation, myo-cardial infarction, stroke, pneumonia, progressive renal insufficiency, acute renal failure, mechanical ventilation over 48 h, surgical site infection, sepsis, unplanned intubation, UTI, or unplanned return to the operating room [Table 8.1]. The authors

Table 8.1 Serious postop-erative morbidity associated with current smoking, alcohol abuse, and hypertension requiring medications

Cardiac arrest requiring CPR
Myocardial infarction
Stroke
Pneumonia
Acute renal failure
Progressive renal insufficiency
Mechanical ventilation
Surgical site infection
Sepsis
UTI
Unplanned intubation
Unplanned return to the operating room

Table 8.2 Preoperative considerations to optimize patient outcomes after neck dissection	Nutritional
	Speech and swallowing
	Thyroid hormone
	Smoking cessation
	Blood thinners
	Social
	Psychology

hypothesized that smoking, alcohol, and hypertension may have been significant due to their direct impact on the physiology of wound healing, tissue viability, and micro-circulation [3].

Given the significant morbidity associated with these frequently observed risk factors in a patient requiring neck dissection, and to optimize long-term outcomes in the patient's form and function, preoperative interventions are warranted regarding the patient's nutrition, smoking/alcohol cessation, and preoperative optimization of medical comorbidities [Table 8.2]. In neck dissection, complications from malnutrition are vast, including wound breakdown, edema, lymphedema, infection, and sepsis. Preoperative serum albumin level has been an independent predictor of surgical outcomes with less surgical complications correlated with normal albumin concentrations [4]. Likewise, Shum et al. studied low prealbumin level being a risk factor for microvascular free flap failure in head and neck reconstruction [5]. Furthermore, similar to the previous findings, in addition to low prealbumin levels, alcohol abuse, smoking history, and hypertension were additional risk factors associated with higher complication rates. Notably, many of these risk factors are influential to one another, such as poor nutrition associated with current alcohol abuse, or smoking increasing the risk of hypertension.

The impact of smoking on patient outcomes cannot be ovestated. With regard to neck dissection, smoking is well known to increase wound breakdown, ensures poor wound healing, and can lead to reactive airway and coughing that lead to a hematoma. Postoperative healing complications occur significantly more often in smokers compared to nonsmokers, as well as in former smokers. However, it is still worthwhile to quit preoperatively, as perioperative smoking cessation has shown to reduce surgical site infections [6]. Even with the known surgical site complications and increased oncologic recurrence rates in head and neck cancer patients who smoke, in a recent study only 53.6% patients stopped smoking after diagnosis or during treatment [7]. Significant smoking cessation education and support is needed to optimize the outcome for neck dissection patients. This can include pamphlets, preoperative surgical optimization team who counsels the patient in smoking cessation, as well as pharmacologic aids by the primary care physicians.

Primary care physicians have multiple unique roles in coordinating care with the surgeon, especially preoperatively. Every year in the United States, approximately 250,000 patients are faced with the challenging situation regarding the periprocedural management of their anticoagulation and antiplatelet medications [8]. In addition to the large number of patients on these medications, it can be challenging for surgeons to be well versed with the many new drugs being developed on an annual basis. Neck dissection and other head and neck surgeries are prone to bleeding complications, and these medications must be properly managed to ensure an optimal outcome for our patients, and prevent these unwanted issues. Cessation and resumption are based on the close relationship that the primary care physician has cultivated with the patient and is based on the interplay between the risk and benefits of anticoagulation. Early cessation can lead to thromboembolic events, and early resumption of these medications can increase the risk of postoperative hemorrhage, hematoma, and possible airway compromise. It is beneficial for surgeons, however, to be aware that the most recent literature recommends that warfarin be resumed 12–24 h after surgery; rivaroxaban, apixaban, and dabigatran can be resumed 2–3 days postoperatively; aspirin and clopidogrel can be resumed 24 h after surgery [9].

A frequently forgotten and underemphasized factor in proper wound healing and recovery is the thyroid function. Unfortunately, even in non-thyroid head and neck cancers managed primarily with surgery and adjuvant radiation, 15% of patients develop hypothyroidism after treatment. In patients that presented for total laryngectomy, neck dissection, and thyroid lobectomy, the incidence is significantly higher at 61% [10]. It is imperative for the patient's thyroid status be investigated and optimized before neck dissection to ensure proper healing and metabolism.

The last preoperative consideration, which will be discussed in further detail during postoperative complications, includes the patient with previous radiation therapy. This patient population has compromised healing capacity, altered anatomy, hyperemic tissue, and often limited cervical extension. With these considerations, incision design that will allow for tension-free closure is very important. If unable to obtain a tension-free closure, consideration for a local or regional flap should be discussed with the patient for closure. Furthermore, given that these patients will be receiving salvage neck dissection after failure of primary chemoradiation, consideration for carotid coverage, and need for healthy distant tissue should be discussed with the patient.

Finally, our goal as a multidisciplinary team caring for patients with oral, head, and neck cancer, is to return the patient to a functional and productive member of the society. The importance of early speech therapy cannot be overemphasized, as it is one of the key outcomes patients designate as high importance in quality of life [11]. The major impact of surgery and potential adjuvant therapy, which can synergistically worsen the patient's speech and swallow function, may be due to poor hyolaryngeal excursion, lymphedema, and/or radiation-induced fibrosis of the neck and associated structures. To offset the impact of the neck dissection and radiation treatment, preoperative speech and language pathologist evaluation is necessary. Numerous studies have demonstrated that performing pretreatment swallowing exercises produce measurable improvements in post-treatment swallowing function in patients [12, 13]. Collaborative multidisciplinary care with a speech-language pathologist is necessary to optimize post-neck dissection functional outcomes.

Intraoperative Complications

Intraoperative complications during neck dissections are usually recognized and can be corrected immediately. Therefore, it is important for the surgeon to be aware of these rare complications to ensure appropriate recognition and treatment can be rendered in a timely manner. These complications are organized as they may be encountered in a sequence of typical neck dissection.

When developing subplatysmal flaps during neck dissections, it is important to plan for the possible tracheostomy. Communication between the tracheostomy site and the neck dissection can lead to tracheal secretions contaminating the neck. This can lead to fistula formation, infection, and hemorrhage from exposed vessels within the neck. This communication may also prevent negative pressure drains from functioning properly, leading to hematoma and seroma formation [14]. Solutions include closing the communication with a local muscle flap (strap or sternocleidomastoid), closing the platysma to the remaining fascia around the communication, and if necessary, using a regional flap (pectoralis major or supraclavicular artery island) for closure.

While removing the fibrofatty tissue, if perforation of the pharynx is detected during surgery, then primary closure is the treatment of choice, when a tension-free closure is possible. In addition to clinical visual detection, a salivary leak may be noted. If concerned and no obvious perforation noted, an Asepto syringe with saline or saline mixed with betadine could be irrigated in the mouth, and the pharynx evaluated for a leak. This region then can be closed primarily, and if closure is not possible, then a local muscle flap may be used for closure, such as the strap muscle, sternocleidomastoid, or regional flaps such as the supraclavicular flap. Of note, if the defect goes undetected and/or is large, and there is a persistent pharyngocutaneous fistula, then a locoregional or free flap may be considered [15]. Placement of nasogastric feeding tube to bypass the pharynx and allow pharyngeal rest is mandatory to prevent saliva contamination of the neck. Postoperatively, it is imperative that the patient's nutrition is advanced slowly, and anti-emetics are used liberally to ensure the patient does not have emesis and breakdown of the pharyngeal closure. Evaluation of the perforation at this juncture can be done with contrast swallow studies, CT scans, or endoscopy. IV antibiotics are required and open drainage may be necessary if perforation persists and is collecting in the neck [15].

Other perforations that may occur are tracheal and/or laryngeal perforations. Intraoperatively, they may be detected at the time of surgery using irrigation to flood the surgical field and monitoring for air bubbles during a Valsalva maneuver. Pinpoint perforations can be challenging to detect, and may not require treatment, especially if the patient is does not require positive pressure ventilation above the glottis. Endotracheal or trans-tracheal ventilation can bypass the perforation and allow closure by secondary intention. If the perforation is easily detected, then occlusion of the perforation with small muscle flap is typically sufficient for closure. Similarly, if positive pressure ventilation is required, then the ETT cuff must be past the perforation [16]. With large perforations, closure with a muscle flap and extended time of intubation may be needed to allow for time to heal. Alternatively, a tracheotomy could be performed to allow time for healing.

Once you are within the region of the carotid sheath, bradycardia induced by carotid manipulation is well described in the literature and is known to occur during neck dissection. It is associated with the baroreceptor reflex from manipulation of the carotid bulb. In addition, bradycardia can be caused by direct vagal stimulation and the trigemino-cardiac reflex. These result in parasympathetic stimulation of the sinoatrial (SA) node resulting in bradycardia and hypotension [17]. These changes in heart rate and blood pressure are usually transient and can immediately be remedied by releasing the pressure on the carotid. However, if it persistent, then anticholinergic medications (glycopyrrolate and/or atropine) may be used to prevent demand-driven ischemia. Chest compressions with ACLS protocol may be required if hemodynamic instability is not improved after use of medications [18].

Stroke due to emboli from carotid manipulation is not common, but it has been described in the literature [19, 20]. Preoperative screening, including patient history and symptoms for significant carotid stenosis, is important. Doppler ultrasonography may be helpful to stratify the risk of a neck dissection in patients with severe carotid stenosis [20]. Intraoperative stroke may lead to changes in respiration and EKG [21, 22]. Often times a stroke is not identified until in the postoperative period. The BE FAST (Balance, Eyes, Face, Arm, Speech, and Time) pneumonic is helpful to identify a stroke patient and urges prompt intervention. If a stroke is suspected, then imaging is needed to confirm, with subsequent thrombolytic therapy or vascular interventions, if warranted. Close monitoring for hematoma formation is necessary with the use of thrombolytic therapy.

An air embolus during a neck dissection is most common after internal jugular vein (IJV) injury [14]. Air embolus causes air to be a space occupier in the vascular lumen, restricting blood flow, resulting in hypoxemia, hypercapnia, cardiac strain arrhythmia, and possible circulatory collapse. A significant air embolus leads to a sudden fall in end-tidal CO_2, which is typically first noticed by the anesthesia team. Treatment involves placing the patient into Trendelenburg and left lateral decubitus position. This positioning allows the air in the heart to be stabilized at the apex of the ventricle, which decreases obstruction of blood flow. Aspiration of the entrapped air with a central venous line and/or open surgery may be required, if the embolus is significant in size. Over time, the air embolus slowly resolves. This process can be sped up with the use of 100% O_2 and hyperbaric oxygen therapy [23]. Prevention of this complication with knowledge of the common etiology and early recognition is the best course of action, rather than treating the complication after the embolus becomes a significant size.

If pneumothorax is suspected intraoperatively, similar to laryngeal/tracheal perforation, the surgical field should be flooded with saline, then it should be confirmed with Valsalva with the patient in Trendelenburg position to detect air bubbles [14]. If a pleural perforation is able to be accessed, then an attempt to close the perforation primarily should be undertaken. If unable to close primarily, then a suction catheter may be placed to decompress the lung, and locoregional tissue can be used to close and obliterate the area. A pig-tail or formal chest tube may still be required if local measures fail to treat the pneumothorax. Postoperative serial chest X-rays are needed to monitor for resolution, and positive pressure ventilation should be avoided [24].

Finally, when performing closure of a neck dissection wound, it must be tension-free. Even in previously non-operated necks, closure can be challenging. Typically, this may be associated with simultaneous free tissue transfer, where the tissue is bulky with a thick subcutaneous fat or large muscular component. Initially, you can attempt to promote wound creep using either 2–0 Vicryl or silk to promote a more passive closure. Flexion of the neck may also be attempted to bring the wound edges into closer proximity. If closure is still not possible, then regional flaps (supraclavicular artery island flap, internal mammary artery perforator, or pectoralis major) can be considered to obtain closure. Additionally, a split thickness skin graft could be considered for covering the muscle component of a free flap. Furthermore, in patients with a history of radiation to the neck, free tissue transfer should be considered to avoid closure under tension (Figs. 8.1–8.4). A common solution, if the flap recipient site is close to the neck, is designing the region of tension near the planned

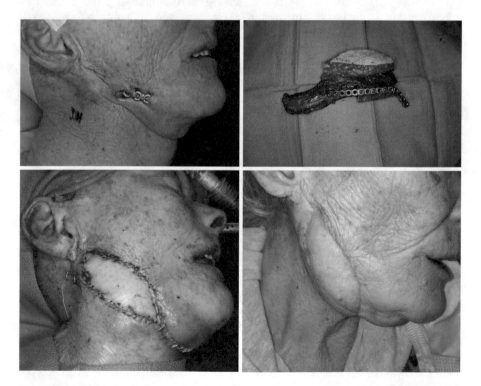

Figs. 8.1–8.4 Patient with a history of neck dissection and radiation therapy. Subsequently, she developed osteoradionecrosis of the right mandible requiring resection and treated with reconstruction plate without bone graft. Two months postoperatively, she presented with exposed mandibular hardware (Fig. 8.1). The patient was taken to OR for fibula free flap with skin paddle for reconstruction of the right mandible and cutaneous defect with the incision incorporated in the neck incision (Fig. 8.2). The patient after inset of fibula and skin paddle sutured to the site of the cutaneous defect (Fig. 8.3). Four-month follow-up shows well-healed skin paddle with no signs of dehiscence (Fig. 8.4)

free flap margin and reconstructing this area with a skin paddle from the free flap [24]. Muscle flaps such as pectoralis major and latissimus dorsi may be used if significant coverage is needed, in conjunction with a split thickness skin graft.

Immediate Postoperative Complications

Although significant care and expertise were employed intraoperatively, vigilance continues to be essential during the immediate postoperative period. The complications encountered in this period can be emergent or very slow to develop and subtle. Prevention continues to be the key with early recognition and treatment leading to decreased morbidity and mortality.

A common complication after neck dissection is the failure of negative pressure drain. Negative pressure drain malfunction ultimately leads to poor drainage, whether from occlusion or lack of an airtight closure. The best prevention for drain malfunction is frequent stripping. The nursing staff should strip the drains frequently, and it should be done by the surgical team as well. If unable to be resolved, it is best to remove the drain, given the risk for infection from a foreign body. In contrast, if there is significant fluid output around the drain, or collection of fluid in the neck, then returning to the OR to replace the drain must be considered. If a drain is not holding suction, the wound needs to be investigated for dehiscence or inadequate closure, especially when an oral closure is involved. If the oral communication has been ruled out, the drain may then be placed on low continuous wall suction, and if able to hold suction, then may continue to monitor on wall suction. If the drain still fails to hold suction, even with low continuous suction, then returning to the OR must be considered to assess closure and place new drain. If a drain is partially pulled out, attempts should be made to make it hold suction again. This can be accomplished by using Tegaderm (3 M, St. Paul, MN) or other occlusive dressing. If a drain is fully pulled out, the wound needs to be monitored closely. If there is continuous drainage or fluid collection within the neck, then a return trip to the OR is warranted to replace the drain.

If a saliva leak is suspected, which can be associated with damage to the parotid tail, or oral communication to the neck, then the JP drain contents should be tested for amylase. If a saliva leak is confirmed, then the oral cavity closure needs to be evaluated to rule out drainage to the neck. If salivary leak continues, for low output drains you may continue to monitor JP drain output over time, with addition of adjunct measures such as scopolamine patch and direct compression of the salivary gland. Injecting salivary glands with botulinum toxin is an additional adjunct that can be considered for low-level output [25]. Once the drain output is at an acceptable level for removal, the drain can be removed and the site is monitored for sialocele, fistula, and infection. If a sialocele forms, then the treatment will require drainage and a compression dressing [26]. If there is a high-volume saliva leak, again an attempt to identify the site of the oral communication should be performed and returning to the OR for closure may be considered, although packing these larger fistulas may also be considered.

Seromas, similar to salivary leak, may be encountered postoperatively. Drainage and application of a compression dressing is typically sufficient for treatment. Drainage can be accomplished with a small incision or needle aspiration. Ultrasound-guided aspiration is a nice adjunct, especially considering the proximity of great vessels. If large, persistent, or suspicious of infection, returning to the OR should be considered for incision and drainage with exploration and drain placement.

If a postoperative pneumothorax is suspected, whether from positive ventilation or from neck dissection, many symptoms and signs present by a development of respiratory or cardiac instability, in addition to loss of breath sounds on the effected side [24]. Prompt recognition and evaluation with a chest X-ray should be done to confirm the pneumothorax [14]. If clinically warranted, needle thoracotomy and decompression of the tension pneumothorax may be necessary, depending on the severity. If a small pneumothorax is found, then no invasive treatment is indicated [27]. If the pneumothorax is causing hemodynamic instability, then thoracostomy tube placement is necessary until resolved. Any pneumothorax should be serially monitored with chest X-rays.

There are also two additional rare postoperative complications associated with deep neck manipulation, especially around the carotid fascia. Oculosympathetic paresis (Horner syndrome) is a recognized complication of neck surgery, with an incidence is 0.5–10%. Surgical implications include neck traction, compression, thermal injuries, and neuropraxia in the carotid sheath [28]. Furthermore, Bernard-Horner's syndrome is caused by damage to sympathetic system, which can be due to thyrocervical venous dilation or damage to the sympathetic nerve trunk, when the plane of dissection is deeper than carotid artery [29]. Many of these require no intervention and supportive care only. However, recognizing the condition, and confirming, obviates the need for exhaustive and expensive workup [28].

Other immediate postoperative complications that the surgeons may encounter include suture abscesses. These nuances typically develop with localized swelling and erythema at the incision line with no evidence of deeper abscess formation. If mild, and abscess formation is questionable, then a course of antibiotics may be acceptable treatment. If abscess formation is obvious, then the best treatment is to sterilize the skin with betadine, locally anesthetize the area, and perform an incision and drainage with removal of the offending suture. The incision and drainage site can then be packed with gauze. Early detection is important for this condition, as significant abscess may develop deep to the skin, before it is visible on the surface.

As discussed in the preoperative section of this chapter, early recognition and optimization of thyroid hormone can pay significant dividends. Checking TSH is important in the postoperative period as hypothyroidism is common in head and neck cancer patients. Hypothyroidism may be the result of the surgery itself, and hypothyroidism in head and neck surgery patients may contribute to poor wound healing, fistula formation, and generalized deterioration. All patients need to be screened for hypothyroidism and treated if necessary [24].

Distant Postoperative Complications

Distant postoperative complications from neck dissections are multifactorial and present with varying timelines. The type of surgical extirpation and reconstruction, exposure to adjuvant chemotherapy and/or radiation, and the patient's nutrition status, in addition to the neck dissection, all play significant roles in the patient's postoperative course.

Head and neck lymphedema is a well-known long-term complication of neck dissections, particularly bilateral neck dissections. Lymphedema may arise due to the disruption of lymphatic drainage, and also due to radiation fibrosis of remaining lymphatic channels. The prevalence of lymphedema is frequently and as high as 90% of head and neck cancer survivors [30]. The significance of lymphedema includes inflammation and tissue fibrosis, and masking of possible recurrence [30]. Thus, continued high index of suspicion for a locoregional recurrence, while performing a thorough head and neck exam, is important to note in the setting of head and neck lymphedema. Multidisciplinary care with speech and language pathologists and physical therapists for lymphedema treatment should be continued postoperatively. In some institutions, lymphedema therapists who devote their practice to lymphedema may be available. Common treatments include manual lymph drainage, use of compression garments, skin care, and exercises of the head and neck. Symptomatic improvement is correlated with adherence to the program regimen and varies depending on extent of surgery and if radiation was required [30]. A 2015 study by Smith and Hucheson et al. showed 60% of patients undergoing lymphedema therapy had a significant decrease in signs and symptoms associated with head and neck lymphedema [31].

Other complications of lymphatic system include the chylous fistula, which are well known and discussed in another chapter. However, not all chyle leaks are through the neck, and can lead to chylothorax and chylous ascites [32, 33]. A particularly unusual lymphatic system complication associated with neck dissection is a lower extremity lymphedema. Raguse et al. reported intraoperative chyle leak controlled with suture ligation, and subsequent return to OR for ligation of the thoracic duct and superior tributary. However, this led to progressive lower extremity lymphedema from the chest to the ankle. A DVT scan was negative, and the lymphedema spontaneously resolved in 2 weeks [34]. In another case associated with bilateral chylothorax, the authors conjectured that an increase in intraluminal pressure of the thoracic duct after ligation can explain lower extremity lymphedema, when no other reasons could be found [32]. Treatment involves leg elevation and compression stockings as first line.

Xerostomia and dysphagia are known long-term complications after head and neck cancer treatment, especially after radiation therapy [35]. Specifically with neck dissection, traditionally, the submandibular gland is excised with level IB lymphadenectomy. Removal of one submandibular gland has been shown to cause some degree of xerostomia, which is compounded with the removal of bilateral submandibular glands [36]. Furthermore, xerostomia is worsened with postoperative radiation therapy, which adversely affects the parotid glands (which produce ~60% of saliva normally) by causing atrophy and further decreasing salivary flow [36]. Submandibular glands can be preserved when performing neck dissections for patients with pT1pN0–1 oral cavity tumors and may be considered to minimize xerostomia [37]. Treatments for xerostomia include hydration, salivary substitutes, and certain toothpastes that may be used for symptomatic relief, while systemic pilocarpine and cevimeline are best for long-term symptomatic improvement [38]. Associated with xerostomia, dysphagia may be exacerbated by a decrease in saliva production as well. However, from a neck dissection, dysphagia may be caused due to iatrogenic injury to vital structures such as hypoglossal nerve and ansa cervicalis during a neck dissection and can be prevented with careful attention to detail. However, a well-executed neck dissection should not in itself be a cause of dysphagia, and a more commonly known sequalae of radiation therapy [38]. Treatment of dysphagia in the setting of neck dissection only includes full workup typically done by speech pathology followed by swallowing exercise and PO intake modifications [39].

There are rare distant complications of neck dissection, which are exacerbated with adjuvant therapy, especially radiation therapy. Chondroradionecrosis (CRN) is a dreaded complication of radiotherapy, which may present months to years after treatment. The incidence of CRN has been reported at 1–5%. CRN is caused primarily by decreased vascularity to the laryngeal cartilage, which leads to ischemia, fibrosis, scarring, and possible tissue death and infection [40]. CRN is seen in both primary and adjuvant radiotherapy. CRN development has been shown to be associated with cartilage invasion by tumor, and ongoing use of both alcohol and smoking. Primary treatment includes tracheotomy and an attempt to halt progression with antibiotics with or without steroids. Hyperbaric oxygen is an additional treatment to consider. Ultimately, if the patient has persistent aspiration and laryngeal dysfunction, then total laryngectomy is indicated [40].

Finally, an odd complication associated with neck dissection and microvascular reconstruction utilizing a venous coupler is coupler dehiscence and exposure through the skin. This is noted with the Synovis GEM Flow Coupler (Synovis MCA, Birmingham, AL) (Fig. 8.5). Most frequently noted in patients with neck dissection and adjuvant radiation, the skin rubs/abuts the plastic coupler, which ultimately can lead to skin necrosis and exposure of the coupler. Anecdotally, if the flap has been inset long enough, the coupler can simply be excised. If not, local wound care and tissue transfer to close the wound over the coupler is necessary. However, significant bleeding may be experienced as well as flap loss, therefore timing since anastomosis, and preoperative imaging such as CT angiogram could be considered before ligation of the vein. Flap loss up to 3 years after free tissue transfer has been reported, especially in the setting of postoperative radiation [41]. Significant bleeding should be prevented by performing the procedure in the operating room, and the surgeon may consider utilizing vessel loops to determine peripheral neovascularization before considering ligation.

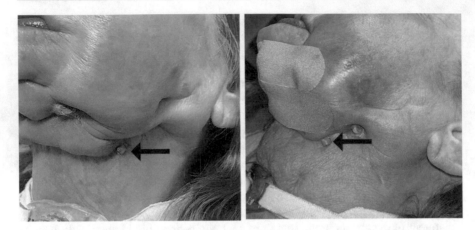

Fig. 8.5 Patient with history of floor of mouth and mandible squamous cell carcinoma who had undergone resection with fibula free flap reconstruction and bilateral neck dissection. She then completed adjuvant radiation. The Synovis GEM Flow Coupler (SynovisMCA, Birmingham, AL) was noticed to be extruding from the skin at a follow-up appointment approximately 1 year after the initial surgery

Conclusion

Neck dissection is a well-described and safe procedure when the patient is optimized during the preoperative period. Intraoperative and immediate postoperative complications have better outcomes if recognized and treated immediately. Long-term, structured patient follow-up and care ensure recognition and proper treatment of late-onset complications.

References

1. Khuri SF, Daley J, Henderson W, et al. National VA surgical quality improvement program. The Department of Veterans Affairs' NSQIP: the first national, validated, outcome-based, risk-adjusted, and peer-controlled program for the measurement and enhancement of the quality of surgical care. Ann Surg. 1998;228(4):491–507.
2. Ma Y, Laitman B, Patel V, et al. Assessment of the NSQIP surgical risk calculator in predicting microvascular head and neck reconstruction outcomes. Head Neck. 2018;160:100–6.
3. Lewis C, Aloia T, Shi W, et al. Development and feasibility of a specialty-specific surgical quality improvement program (NSQIP): the head and neck-reconstructive surgery NSQIP. JAMA Oto. 2016;142(4):321–7.
4. Gibbs J, Cull W, Henderson W, et al. Preoperative serum albumin level as a predictor of operative mortality and morbidity. JAMA Surg. 1999;134(1):36–42.
5. Shum J, Markiewicz M, Park E, et al. Low prealbumin level is a risk factor for microvascular free flap failure. J Oral Maxillofac Surg. 2014;72:169–77.
6. Sorensen L. Wound healing and infection in surgery: the clinical impact of smoking and smoking cessation: a systematic review and meta-analysis. JAMA Surg. 2012;147(4):373–83.

7. Chan Y, Irish J, Wood S, et al. Smoking cessation in patients diagnosed with head and neck cancer. Head Neck. 2004;33(2):75–81.
8. Spyropoulos AC, Douketis JD. How I treat anticoagulated patients undergoing elective procedure or surgery. Blood. 2012;120:2954–62.
9. Jethwa A, Khariwala S. When should therapeutic anticoagulation be restarted following major head and neck surgery? Laryngoscope. 2017;128(5):1025–6.
10. Sinard R, Tobin E, Mazzaferri E, et al. Hypothyroidism after treatment for nonthyroid head and neck cancer. Arch Otolaryngol Head Neck Surg. 2000;126:652–7.
11. Kim R, Burkes J, Williams F. Predicting quality of life (QoL) of oral cancer. In: Kademani D, editor. Improving outcomes in oral cancer: a clinical and translational update: Springer International Publishing: Switzerland; 2020. p. 181–9.
12. Carroll WR, Locher JL, Canon CL, Bohannon IA, McColloch NL, Magnuson JS. Pretreatment swallowing exercises improve swallow function after chemoradiation. Laryngoscope. 2008;118:39–43.
13. Roe JW, Ashforth KM. Prophylactic swallowing exercise for patients receiving radiotherapy for head and neck cancer. Curr Opin Otolaryngol Head Neck Surg. 2011;19:144–9.
14. Kerawala CJ, Heliotos M. Prevention of complications in neck dissection. Head Neck Oncol. 2009;1(35):1–6.
15. Busoni M, Deganello A, Gallo O. Pharyngocutaneous fistula following total laryngectomy: analysis of risk factors, prognosis, and treatment modalities. ACTA Otorhinolaryngol. 2015;35:400–5.
16. Satyadas T, Nasir N, Erel E, Mudan S. Iatrogenic tracheal rupture: a novel approach to repair and review of the literature. J Trauma. 2003;54:369–71.
17. Tarabanic C, Abt N, Osborn H. Intraoperative cardiac arrest etiologies in head and neck surgery: a compregensive review. Head Neck. 2018;40:1299–304.
18. Higuchi H, Ishii M, Nakatsuka H, Maeda S, Morita K, Miyawaki T. Sudden cardiac arrest in head and neck surgery: a case report. J Anesth. 2010;24:146–7.
19. Cramer J, Patel U, Maas M, Samant S, Smith S. Is neck dissection associated with an increased risk of postoperative stroke? Otolaryngol Head Neck Surg. 2017;157(2):226–32.
20. Thompson S, Mckinnon G, Ghali W. Perioperative stroke occurring in patients who undergo neck dissection for head and neck cancer: unanswered questions. Can J Surg. 2003;46(5):332–4.
21. Rochester C, Mohsenin V. Respiratory complications of stroke. Semin Respir Crit Care Med. 2002;22(3):248–60.
22. Wira C, Rivers E, Martinez-Capolino C, Silver B, Iyer G, Sherwin R, Lewandowski C. Cardiac complications in acute ischemis stroke. West J Emerg Med. 2001;12(4):414–20.
23. Gordy S, Rowell S. Vascular air embolism. Int J Crit Illn Inj Sci. 2013;3(1):73–6.
24. Genden E, Ferlito A, Shaha A, Talmi Y, Robbins T, Rhys-Evans P, Rinaldo A. Complications of neck dissection. Acta Otolaryngol. 2003;123:795–801.
25. Maharaj S, Mungul S, Laher A. Botulinum toxin A is an effective therapeutic tool for the management of parotid sialocele and fistula: a systematic review. Laryngoscope Investig Otolaryngol. 2020;5:37–45.
26. Kudva A, Carriappa K, Kamath A, Chithra A. Compression dressing using dental impression compound for conservative management of sialocele. J Maxillofac Oral Surg. 2016;15(4):555–7.
27. Huang Y, Huang H, Li Q, Browning R, Parrish S, Turner F, Zarogoulidis K, Kougioumtzi I, Dryllis G, Kioumis I, Pitsiou G, Machairiotis N, Katsikogiannis N, Courcoutsakis N, Madesis A, Diplaris K, Karaiskos T, Zarogoulidis P. Approach of the treatment for pneumothorax. J Thorac Dis. 2014;6:s416–20.
28. Mumtaz S, Parrish J, Singh M. Oculosympathetic paresis after selective neck dissection: a "distant" complication. Oral Oncol. 2018;79:78–9.
29. Bucci T, Califano L. Bernard-Horner's syndrome: unusual complication after neck dissection. JOMS. 2008;66(4):833.

30. Gutierrez C, Karni R, Naqvi S, Aldrich M, Zhu B, Morrow R, Sevick-Muraca E, Rasmussen J. Head and neck lymphedema: treatment response to single and multiple sessions of advanced pneumatic compression therapy. Otolaryngol Head Neck Surg. 2019;160(4):622–6.
31. Smith B, Hutcheson K, Little L, Skoracki R, Rosenthal D, Lai S, Lewin F. Lymphedema outcomes in patients with head and neck cancer. Otolaryngol Head Neck Surg. 2015;152(2):284–91.
32. Busquets J, Rullan P, Trinidad-Pinedo J. Bilateral chylothorax after neck dissection. Otolaryngol Head Neck Surg. 2004;130(4):492–5.
33. Majdalany B, El-Haddad G. Contemporary lymphatic interventions for post-operative lymphatic leaks. Transl Androl Urol. 2020;9:s104–13.
34. Raguse J, Pfitzmann R, Bier J, Klein M. Lower-extremity lymphedema following neck dissection – an uncommon complication after cervical ligation of the thoracic duct. Oral Oncol. 2007;43:835–7.
35. Bressan V, Stevanin S, Bianchi M, Aleo G, Bagnasco A, Sasso L. The effects of swallowing disorders, dysgeusia, oral mucositis and xerostomia on nutritional status, oral intake and weight loss in head and neck cancer patients: a systemic review. Cancer Treat Rev. 2016;45:105–19.
36. Jaguar G, Lima E, Kowalski L, Pellizon A, Carvalho A, Alves F. Impact of submandibular gland excision on salivary gland function in head and neck cancer patients. Oral Oncol. 2010;46:349–54.
37. Subramaniam N, Balasubramanian D, Reddy R, Rathod P, Murthy S, Vidhyadharan S, Thankappan K, Iyer S. Determinants of level Ib involvement in oral squamous cell carcinoma and implications for submandibular gland-sparing neck dissection. Int J Oral Maxillofac Surg. 2018;47:1507–10.
38. Mercadante V, Hamad A, Lodi G, Porter S, Fedele S. Interventions for the management of radiotherapy-induced xerostomia and hyposalivation: a systematic review and meta-analysis. Oral Oncol. 2017;66:64–74.
39. Cantemir S, Laubert A. Diagnostics and therapy of dysphagia. ENT. 2017;65:347–56.
40. Gessert T, Britt C, Maas A, Wieland A, Harari P, Hartig G. Chondroradionecrosis of the larynx: 24-year University of Wisconsin experience. Head Neck. 2017;39:1189–94.
41. Moolenburgh S, van Huizum M, Hofer S. DIEP-flap failure after pedicle division three years following transfer. Br J Plast Surg. 2005;58:1000–3.

Index

A
Abscess, 49, 85, 87, 88, 151
Afatinib, 133, 134
American College of Surgeons Nation
      Surgical Quality Improvement
      Program® (NISQIP®), 144
American Society of Anesthesiologists
      (ASA), 50
Angiosome-based approach, 25, 26
Anterior midline neck, 26
Anterior neck muscles, 26
Anterolateral thigh (ALT) free flap, 113
Antibiotic prophylaxis, 51–53
Antibiotics, 125
Apron incision, 33–35, 40, 81

B
Balance, Eyes, Face, Arm, Speech, and Time
      (BE FAST), 148
Balloon test occlusion (BTO), 120
Bernard-Horner's syndrome, 151
Blood supply, 24
Brachial plexus, 105, 106

C
Carotid artery, 118, 119, 124
Carotid blowout syndrome (CBS), 55, 56,
      85, 86, 89
  acute, 89, 90
  incidence of, 86
  pathophysiology, 87
  type I, 85, 88
  type II, 85, 88
  type III, 86, 88
Central Skin flap necrosis, 65
Cervical lymph nodes, 5, 6
Cervical plexus, 101, 104–106

Cervical sympathetic chain, 108
Cetuximab, 133
Cevimeline, 153
Chondroradionecrosis (CRN), 153
Chyle leak
  activity modification, 71
  complications, 64–67
  conservative management, 71
  diagnosis of, 65, 66, 68
  diet modification, 71
    elemental formula, 72
    MCT, 71, 72
    TPN, 72
  immediate intraoperative management, 68
    identification and ligation, 68, 69
    local flaps, 69, 70
  intraoperative valsalva maneuver, 66, 67
  invasive and surgical treatment
    percutaneous transabdominal lymphatic
      access, 74, 75
    surgical exploration, 75
    thoracoscopic ligation of thoracic
      duct, 76
    transcervical thoracic duct puncture, 75
  pharmacological methods
    etilefrine, 74
    orlistat, 74
    somatostatin, 73
  postoperative diagnosis of, 70
  postoperative management, 71
  risk factors of, 63
  wound care
    negative pressure wound therapy, 73
    pressure dressing, 72, 73
    suction drains, 72
Clindamycin, 51, 52
Closed surgical drains (CSD), 43
Combined Positive Score (CPS), 133
Composite resection, 113

Comprehensive neck dissection, 6, 9
Conservative management
    chyle leak, 71
    skin incision complications
        CSD, 43
        NPWT, 41–43
        wet to dry therapy, 41, 42

D
Deeper dermis, 23
Dehiscence, 35, 39, 40
Delayed wound healing, 39
Dermal-subdermal plexus, 26
Diet modification, chyle leak
    elemental formula, 72
    MCT, 71, 72
    TPN, 72
Disease-free survival (DFS), 18
Disease-specific survival (DSS), 18
Distant postoperative complications, 152–154
Durant's maneuver, 83
Dysphagia, 152

E
Elastic fibers, 24
Epidermis, 23
Etilefrine, 74
EXTREME trial, 133

F
Fibular free flap, 113
Functional neck dissection (FND), 5, 6, 10,
    112, 117

G
Great auricular nerve, 104, 105

H
Habit modification, 38
Head and neck surgery, 55
Hyperbaric oxygen, 153
Hypertrophic scars, 29
Hypoglossal nerve, 104

I
Immediate postoperative complications,
    150, 151
Infectious complications

antibiotic prophylaxis, 51–53
carotid blowout, 55, 56
definitions, epidemiology and risk
    factors, 49, 50
financial burden, 56
management, 54
mitigation, 53, 54
necrotizing SSI, 55
outcomes, 55
pathogens, 50, 51
Internal jugular blowout (IJB), 86, 87
    pathophysiology, 87
    presentation and management, 88
Internal jugular vein (IJV), 112, 113, 115–117
Intracranial pressure (ICP), 116
Intraoperative complications, 147–150
Intraoral soft tissue defect, 113

K
Klebsiella pneumoniae, 50

L
Length of stay (LOS), 56
Lingual nerve, 104
Lip-split incision, 34
Lower lateral neck, 26
Lymphatic system
    anatomy of thoracic duct, 60, 61
    drainage patterns of anatomic
        subsites, 61, 62
    embryology, 59, 60
Lymphedema, 152

M
MacFee incision, 30–31, 115
Marginal mandibular branch of the facial
    nerve, 122–124
Marginal mandibular nerve (MMN),
    97–100, 124
Medium chain triglyceride (MCT), 71, 72
Melanocytes, 24
Merkel cell, 24
Methicillin-resistant *Staphylococcus aureus*
    (MRSA), 51
Mid lateral neck, 26
Modified Blair parotid incision, 33
Modified radical neck dissection (MRND), 5,
    6, 32, 111, 112, 114, 115
    chyle complications, 116
    indication, 114
    nerve complications

marginal mandibular branch of the
    facial nerve, 122–124
phrenic nerve, 125
SAN, 120–122
vagus nerve, 124, 125
type I, 6, 9, 15
type II, 6
type III, 6
vascular complications, 116–120
Modified Schobinger's incision, 32
Morbidity, 144, 145, 150
Mortality, 150
Multidisciplinary care, 146, 152
Myocutaneous flap, 119, 120

N
National Cancer Database, 16
National Comprehensive Cancer Network
    (NCCN) guidelines, 128
Neck dissections, 149
    cervical lymph nodes and
        classification, 5, 6
    comprehensive neck dissections, for
        clinically positive neck, 9
    distant postoperative complications,
        152, 153
    history, 1–5
    immediate postoperative complications,
        150, 151
    indications and outcomes, 15–18
    intraoperative complications, 147–150
    preoperative considerations, 143–146
    selective neck dissections, for clinically
        negative neck
        functional neck dissection, 10
        supraomohyoid neck dissection,
            11, 13, 14
    skin incision complications (see Skin
        incisions)
    vascular complications in (see Vascular
        complications)
Necrotizing fasciitis, 55
Negative pressure wound therapy (NPWT),
    41–43, 73, 116
Nerve supply, 24
Neural complications
    brachial plexus, 105, 106
    cervical plexus, 105
    cervical sympathetic chain, 108
    great auricular nerve, 104, 105
    lingual nerve/hypoglossal nerves, 104
    MMN, 97–100
    phrenic nerve, 106

SAN, 100–103
superior laryngeal nerve, 107, 108
vagus nerve, 106, 107
Nivolumab, 133, 134
N staging, 126
Nutritional status/diet modification, 37–38

O
Occult metastases, 64
Occult neck disease, 1, 5, 13, 15
Octreotide, 73, 116
Oral/head and neck cancer, neck dissections,
    see Neck dissections
Orlistat, 74

P
Pacinian corpuscles, 24
Palliative care, 134
Parenteral antibiotics, 51
Percutaneous transabdominal lymphatic
    access, 74, 75
Perioperative glycemic control, 51
Phrenic nerve, 106, 125
Pilocarpine, 153
Polytetrafluoroethylene (PTFE) grafts, 119
Postoperative infection rates, 125
Postoperative pneumothorax, 151
Preoperative lymphoscintigraphy, 17
Primary care physicians, 145
Prophylactic antibiotics, 56

R
Radiation therapy, 149, 153
Radical neck dissection (RND), 4, 6, 111–113
    chyle complications, 116
    indication, 114
    nerve complications
        marginal mandibular branch of the
            facial nerve, 122–124
        phrenic nerve, 125
        SAN, 120–122
        vagus nerve, 124, 125
    vascular complications, 116–120
Recurrent neck disease, 127
    palliative care, 134
    reirradiation, 130–132
    salvage surgery, 129, 130
    systemic therapy, 132–134
    workup and diagnosis, 127–129
Regional flap, 146, 147, 149
Reirradiation, 130–132

Right modified neck dissection, 113
Right neck tumor, 80
Right pharyngectomy, 113
Right posterior maxillectomy, 113
Right radical neck dissection, 113
Right retromolar trigone, 113
Right segmental mandibulectomy with
        disarticulation, 113

S
Saliva leak, 150
Salvage surgery, 129, 130
Saphenous vein, 119
Scalene muscles, 26
Schobinger incision, 32, 33
Selective neck dissection (SND), 112
        functional neck dissection, 10
        supraomohyoid neck dissection, 11, 13, 14
Septocutaneous arteries, 25
Seromas, 151
Single photon emission computer tomography
        (SPECT), 120
Single transverse incision, 31
Sinoatrial (SA) node, 148
Skin appendages, 24
Skin flap necrosis, 35, 64, 65
Skin incisions
        aging, 28
        designs, 30
                apron incision, 33, 34
                MacFee incision, 30–31
                Schobinger incision, 32
        flap tension, 26, 27
        flap undermining, 27
        general skin physiology, 25
        histological layers
                epidermis and dermis, 23, 24
                neurovascular supply, 24, 25
        keloids/hypertrophic scars, surgical
                management of, 45
        management of skin incision
                complications, 39
                closed surgical drains, 43
                habit modification, 38
                medical optimization, 39
                negative pressure wound therapy, 41–43
                nutritional status/diet
                        modification, 37–38
                prevention, 36
                surgical planning/technique, 39
                wet to dry therapy, 41, 42
        risk factors, 35, 36

sharp/surgical debridement, 44
skin flap design and blood supply, 25, 26
wound healing, 28, 29
Somatostatin (SS), 73
Spinal accessory nerve (SAN), 4, 100–103,
        115, 120–122
Squamous cell carcinoma, 154
Staphylococcus aureus, 50
Sternocleidomastoid muscle, 2, 69, 70, 112,
        113, 115, 120, 121
Submandibular gland, 152
Submaxillary gland, 10
Subplatysmal flaps, 123, 124, 147
Superficial epidermis, 23
Superficial femoral artery (SFA) grafts, 119
Superior laryngeal nerve, 107, 108
Superselective neck dissection, 17
Supraomohyoid neck dissection (SOHND), 2,
        5, 6, 11, 13–16, 18, 62
Surgical Risk Calculator (SRC), 144
Surgical site infection (SSI), 49, 54
        definition, 49
        5-year survival rate, 55
        incidence of, 52
        mitigation of, 53
        necrotizing SSI, 55
Syndrome of inappropriate antidiuretic
        hormone secretion (SIADH), 117
Synovis GEM Flow Coupler, 153, 154
Systemic therapy, 132–134

T
Thermoregulation, 25
Total parenteral nutrition (TPN), 72
Transcervical thoracic duct puncture, 75
T-staging, 126

U
Upper aerodigestive tract, 111, 125, 126
Upper lateral neck, 26

V
Vagus nerve, 106, 107, 124, 125
Vascular complications
        carotid blowout syndrome, 85, 86
        concomitant neck dissection, free flaps
                with, 91, 92
        early postoperative complications, 83, 84
        internal jugular vein blow-out, 86, 87
        pathophysiology, 87

presentation and management, 87, 88
intra-operative vascular
      complications, 81–83
late postoperative complications, 89–91
preoperative considerations, 80, 81
RND and MRND, 116–120

W
Wet to dry therapy, 41, 42

Wound care, chyle leak
   negative pressure wound therapy, 73
   pressure dressing, 72, 73
   suction drains, 72
Wound healing, 28, 29
Wound VAC Versflo technologies, 43

X
Xerostomia, 152, 153

Printed in the United States
by Baker & Taylor Publisher Services